BREAK THROUGH

6 Weeks to Demolish Diet Culture Strongholds

CAROL BEVIL and ALEX BRIGHAM

Published in Birmingham, Alabama by Fuel
Your Body, Feed Your Soul, LLC.

Unless otherwise noted, Scripture quotations are taken from
the Holy Bible, New International Version. Copyright 2015 by
Zondervan, All rights reserved worldwide. www.zondervan.com
The "niv' and "new international version" are trademarks registered
in the United States Patent and Trademark Office by Biblica, Inc.

"Do not be conformed to this world, but be transformed by the renewal of your mind, that by testing you may discern what is the will of God, what is good and acceptable and perfect."

ROMANS 12:2

CONTENTS

WELCOME

HUMBLE BEGINNINGS.
GREAT REWARDS

"Behold. I am doing a new thing: Now it springs forth. Do you not perceive it? I will make a way in the wilderness and rivers in the desert." Isaiah 43:19

Welcome to day one of what can be a stepping stone to freedom for the rest of your life. Freedom from food obsession, from being uncomfortable and at war with your body. Freedom from planning your life around food or from letting your life dictate your health.

Freedom from worldly trends and enemy strongholds that have twisted honoring your body into the false idols of: diet culture, lifestyles, wellness, and self-reliant willpower.

Gone are the days of white-knuckling your way through the day, being "good" and sticking to the meal plan. Now are the days of peace within and joy throughout. Now is the time to walk away from the world's ashes of seeking Tuesday transformation and begin seeking true, lasting transformation in your relationship with food and body image:

> "Do not conform to the patterns of this world, but be transformed by the renewing of your mind. Then you will be able to test and approve what God's will is -- his good, pleasing and perfect will." Romans 12:2

What if we told you that, having been designed by the Creator, you innately know what your body needs to not only survive, but to thrive? What if we told you that we have all been intentionally manipulated into believing otherwise? What if we told you diet culture makes an overwhelming profit by selling you deceit to set you up to fail. And, when you inevitably fail, you are told it is your fault: your life imprisoned in the stronghold of shame.

What if we told you God wants so much more for you than a life battling the stronghold of diet culture. Your body was beautifully and intelligently designed to support itself using the fuel that God provided for us in His wisdom. (Genesis 1:29, 9:3; Mark 7:19). The next six weeks are not a diet plan. This is a journey to reconnect with the truth about our God intended relationship with food and body image.

In the next six weeks, our prayer is the enemy's schemes, slickly marketed as wellness by diet culture, are brought into light, you rediscover the beauty of your body and know it can be trusted, and false idols and strongholds are demolished by seeking God first even in this area of your life. When you surrender to God's truth, turning from self-reliance and worldly gurus, you receive "all the things" and experience the fruit of the Spirit:

> "Love, joy, peace, patience, kindness, goodness, faithfulness, gentleness, and self-control." Galatians 5:22-23.

CAROL + ALEX

PROGRAM OVERVIEW

Each week we will introduce two transformation habits. One to nourish your flesh: Fuel Your Body. One to nurture your spirit: Feed Your Soul.

| FUEL YOUR BODY

The Fuel habits are focused on building a solid foundation so that your body is well-nourished. A well-nourished body is a body that's hunger cues can be trusted and one where cravings are diminished. A well fueled body works for you rather than against you and it releases you from worrying about food. Once the foundation is strong, you develop a relationship of trust with your body. You make choices based on hunger or situation. Choices that are mindful; rather than, being dictated by external diet culture that peddles in fear, false food guilt, and the stronghold of shame. God gave us good things to eat and designed a body with intelligent cues. When we cling to His truth for nourishment, as in all things, we reap the fruit of the Spirit. Truly, with God we are more than conquerors over the enemy's strongholds.

Our six foundational fuel habits for a well-nourished body:

Thirst No More: Sufficient Hydration
Every Seed Bearing Plant: Vegetables & Fruit
Recognizing Fullness
Every Moving Thing: Protein
Manna: Carbohydrates
Fats of the Land: Fat

God's Transformations are Eternal

| FEED YOUR SOUL

The Soul habits are designed to reveal our focus in our relationship with food and our body. Is our focus inward to self and horizontal to the world? Or, is our relationship with food and our body a vertical one, with eyes fixed on the kingdom? In other words, the soul habits, we pray, are designed to reveal and convict. We want to shift your focus from self-reliance and worldly gurus to Spirit empowered and God dependent. Our mindset around food and body has been conformed to the pattern of this world; our desire to conform has caused us to wander from God's protection and blessings in this arena. God's greatest desire is that we draw near to Him. He wants us to know his will for our life so that we can be seed planters and kingdom light bearers. Anything that pulls our focus from God, including anxiety and worry about food and our bodies, diminishes our ability to know his will and fulfill our kingdom purpose. We pray the Soul Habits are the foundation to seeking first the kingdom in this area of your life. We know in our weakness, His power is made strong. We know the Holy Spirit is your helper and will renew your mind. We know through Christ, alone, all things are possible. How do we know? The Bible tells us so. Fix your eyes on Jesus. You will be transformed: from imprisoned in diet culture strongholds to the fullness, freedom, and peace of God.

Our six foundational soul habits to renew your mind:

Giving Thanks
Spirit Empowerment: Filling the Want
In All Your Ways
Jesus. Jesus. Jesus.
Enemy Strongholds
From Fear to Peace

| AT THE KING'S TABLE

> "A person standing alone can be attacked and defeated, but two can stand back-to-back and conquer. Three are even better, for a triple-braided cord is not easily broken." Ecc 4:12

In addition to our two Transformation Habits, each week we include a Bible Study to deepen your roots in God's truth and His desire for your life. We pray, if possible, you gather with others and take a seat at the King's Table, the place where all things are possible. Throughout the Bible, we learn how God values the strengthening and refining power of fellowship. Our prayer, together we demolish diet culture strongholds and sharpen one another. Of course, should you choose to walk through Break Through without peers you are never alone. God is always near. At the King's Table is a sweet time to be uplifted, encouraged, and strengthened through God's Word. Precious time with your Heavenly Father.

| TO DO SOMETHING NEW

We begin with THIRST NO MORE: Sufficient Hydration and GIVE THANKS. Break Through is designed to set you on a path that is Spirit led with Jesus, its goal. If at the end of each week, entrenched enemy strongholds are exposed: SLOW YOUR ROLL. Take the necessary time to feel confident that you are mindfully incorporating both habits and that any false guilt that leads to shame (this is never from God) is rejected! A healthy relationship with food and body has no finish line; it is a daily practice. The ultimate goal is not a superficial, temporary scale-win, but to put on the full armor of God so that you honor your body without falling prey to the enemy's schemes: turning good things like health and wellness into false idols. The ultimate goal is to trade in the world's ashes for the abundant beauty and joyful freedom that can only come from God. The ultimate goal is that through Christ you demolish every enemy stronghold that draws you away from God's truth about Him and about yourself. You have believed lies about your food and body relationships for years. The defining attribute of a stronghold is its recurring pattern: despite its life-draining destructiveness you keep returning to it. Your worth is not found in the mirror or on a scale. Your worth is not tied to your performance and your ability to diet. Rather, your worth was settled on the Cross. You are of such worth to God, He gave His only Son. He is patient. He is faithful. His love is steadfast. His grace is sufficient. It is more than ok to BE STILL and get to the root of your strongholds by prayerfully surrendering them to God. Meditate on His truth so that your mind is renewed and your strongholds demolished.

> "For freedom Christ has set us free; stand firm therefore, and do not submit again to a yokc of slavery." Galatians 5:1

STRONGHOLDS

God's plan for your life is to demolish spiritual strongholds. Often, however, we are not aware of the strongholds we battle. The enemy is sly. He deceives by using our insecurities, false guilt, and pride to construct strongholds that draw us far from the protection and truth of God which, then, further fortifies them in our lives. Deception is not the enemy's only weapon in constructing strongholds that draw you away from God. He also twists and distorts. The source of strongholds isn't confined to just your broken places or wounds. Your strongholds often stem from good pursuits like wellness. Whatever the source, spiritual strongholds are always built of lies. Lies that diminish your trust in, and weaken your relationship with, Jesus. Lies that distort the truth about your worth to God. Lies that shift your focus from the Kingdom to faith in self or the world.

Throughout this journey you will become aware of and convicted to strongholds in your life that keep you from peace in your relationship with food and your body. The enemy has used diet culture to take your thoughts captive and imprison you in the strongholds of: fear, self-reliance, willpower, false guilt, worldly wisdom,and shame (to name just a few). To identify your strongholds as you surrender this area of your life to Jesus know that strongholds often reveal themselves as a recurring pattern. A recurring pattern that doesn't produce the fruit of the spirit, but rather leaves you feeling as if it is a constant struggle from which you can not break free. To become aware of and be convicted to strongholds in your relationship with food and your body, ask yourself if you are seeking the kingdom first or looking to your own strength and worldly gurus. When strongholds are exposed, take them to the Cross.

The good news: God did not leave you to battle alone. In 2 Corinthians 10:3-4, Paul addresses the battle with spiritual strongholds:

> "For though we live in the world, we do not wage war as the world does. The weapons we fight with are not the weapons of the world. On the contrary, they have divine power to demolish strongholds."

During the next 6 weeks, we pray Break Through helps you "demolish arguments and every pretension" of every diet culture's stronghold. We pray you seek God's truth first in this area of your life and fully surrender to it. We know, when you do, not only will He demolish your strongholds so that you experience the fruit of the Spirit in your relationship with food and your body, He will renew your mind and transform your life.

"May the God of hope fill you with all joy and peace as you trust in him, so that you may overflow with hope by the power of the Holy Spirit."

Romans 15:13

THE JOURNEY BEGINS

RELEASING THE OLD

"Behold, I am doing a new thing; now it springs forth, do you not perceive it? I will make a way in the wilderness and rivers in the desert." Isaiah 43:19

This is the first week of learning new things and releasing old habits that haven't served you well.

Even though you know the end destination of this journey is freedom from diet culture strongholds, freedom from false food guilt and body shame, nutrition independence through a renewed mind, it can still be unnerving to go down a road that so few choose to travel.

You'll be asked to ditch dieting and all diet thinking. You'll be asked to remove labels from food like "good" and "bad." You'll have to confront every enemy falsehood that has built faulty thinking patterns about food and your body. You'll be asked to stand firm against those around you that cling to diet culture. It may feel like riding a bike without training wheels or bowling without the bumpers up for the first time, but we promise that you will learn.

This is a new thing that you are doing now. It's new for you and new for the vast majority of our society. You will run into friction, both from others and from yourself. You will stumble and "mess up." But all of that is both expected and welcome. If it weren't for friction and obstacles, how would you grow stronger in Christ? If it weren't for mess ups, how would you learn? Remember all stumbles and obstacles are for your good when rooted in a desire to discern God's truth.

| LEADER-LED DISCUSSION:

- Hesitation is as natural as excitement when beginning any new journey in life. Discuss hesitations about beginning Break Through as well as excitement.
- Journal diet culture strongholds that you want to demolish and where you hope this journey leads.
- God is the God of our everything - food and body included. Discuss what that means to the group in the current moment and what that could mean for them in the future.

RELEASING THE OLD

"... to put off your old self, which belongs to your former manner of life and is corrupt through deceitful desires, and to be renewed in the spirit of your minds, and to put on the new self, created after the likeness of God in true righteousness and holiness." Ephesians 4:22-24

Putting off the old and putting on the new. If you're like most, this isn't your first attempt to put off the old. Did you know that one of the biggest obstacles to achieving lasting change is understanding what exactly the "old self" is?

More times than not we point the finger at the wrong suspects. In trying to lose weight we gravitate towards blaming a certain food (carbs, fat, sugar, etc) or our inability to have enough willpower to say no. What if we told you that those things aren't the "old" that needs putting off? Those are strongholds.

What we've found to be true 100% of the time is that the attitudes we hold in our minds towards food and body are the "old" that need to be put off. It's the fear of food, the complacency with convenience, the belief that willpower is the solution, the desire to fit a predetermined mold, the end goal of aesthetics and not health, and so many more ideas/ attitudes that need to be put off.

And so that raises the question - what is the "new?" As with everything, the answer to this is found in the pages of the Bible: receiving all blessings and nourishment with a heart of thanksgiving, choosing to walk the narrow path of self-control with a heart bent towards grace and forgiveness, the willingness to labor for the harvest to come, the understanding that we have been molded in the likeness of God, and that to bring His name glory through a life lived in the pursuit of the Kingdom is the noblest pursuit.

> "Do not be conformed to this world, but be transformed by the renewal of your mind, that by testing you may discern what is the will of God, what is good and acceptable and perfect."
> Romans 12:2

| LEADER-LED DISCUSSION:

- What is the old? What desires and motivations influenced the "old?"
- We've all tried to change in the past. What were some challenges you faced in previous attempts to change?
- If you could create a new self completely from scratch, molded after the image of God, what would that new person look like? Think like? Speak like? Act like?
- "To be renewed in the spirit of your minds..." Break Through is founded on the idea that renewing the mind must happen first in order to demolish the strongholds that keep us from lasting transformation. Discuss what that means to the group.

"Behold, I am doing a new thing; now it springs forth, do you not perceive it? I will make a way in the wilderness and rivers in the desert."

Isaiah 43:19

WEEK 1
TRANSFORMATION
HABITS

FUEL YOUR BODY
THIRST NO MORE
SUFFICIENT HYDRATION
FEED YOUR SOUL
GIVE THANKS

THIRST NO MORE: SUFFICIENT HYDRATION

> "With joy you will draw water from the wells of salvation." Isaiah 12:3

Water is the essence of life. Water is often referred to as a restorative, cleansing and life-giving substance in the Bible. It has always represented vitality to us and to all living things. So why, then, has it become an after-thought for the majority of people today?

Hydration affects everything in the body, including:

- Digestion and absorption of nutrients
- Transportation and filtration of waste
- Transportation of oxygen in the blood
- Lubrication of mucous membranes
- Temperature regulation
- Muscular contractions
- Cognitive function
- Integrity of skin
- Weight management/Utilization of energy

It's no secret that drinking water is one of the first and simplest things you can do when trying to lose weight or body fat. We aren't diving into that topic, because this isn't ABOUT weight loss. We aren't reinforcing diet culture falsehoods such as: drink water to suppress hunger. Losing unhealthy weight for good (not disliked) results from a well-nourished body and a spirit of self-control. It is never the result of restriction, elimination, or the misguided idea that water is an appetite suppressant or a distraction from hunger. Sufficient hydration is ABOUT gaining life, vitality, understanding your body's design, and clarity of mind. Water is a gift, one that purifies and heals. It is necessary for both our physical and spiritual health. Sufficient hydration is about honoring your body.

HOW MUCH WATER DO YOU NEED?

As little as a 2% loss
of body fluid can lead
to a decrease in mental
and physical function.

The typical recommended goal of baseline water intake is half your bodyweight in ounces. So, if you weigh 150 pounds you need 75 ounces of water each day as your starting amount.

Then, for each of the following you need to add an additional 8 ounces (one glass) of water to your starting amount:

- For every alcoholic beverage you drink
- For every high sodium content food or meal
- For every 30 minutes of exercise, indoors
- For every 20 minutes of exercise, outdoors (add additional 4 ounces in heat of summer)
- For any illness that includes increased body temperature, vomiting, frequent urination or diarrhea (please consult your physician to make certain you are hydrating sufficiently)

Whew! That is a lot of water! You can see how the amount you need each day could start to add up quickly and become overwhelming. Understand that the above are a guide to give you an idea of your estimated daily needs. However, in typical recommendations it is often forgotten that we get quite a bit of water from the foods we eat. A well-balanced diet can supply 20% of our water needs. So, for our example: a 150 pound individual baseline goal from fluid water reduces to 60 ounces because 15 ounces comes from food alone. Water intake is not a fixed amount and ultimately must work in concert with your lifestyle demands. Don't become overwhelmed or fixated on water. Just be aware and mindful.

| HOW TO GET YOUR OUNCES IN

If you are not hydrating sufficiently or barely hydrating, gradually increase your water intake until your thirst is quenched and you are near or at baseline. Yes, we know what most of you are thinking:

YOU WILL HAVE TO PEE. When you drink water the body filters it through its system and excretes it; it's part of your beautiful, efficient design. However, if you gradually increase each day you will find it much easier to adapt and give your body time to adjust. As well, you will reconnect to your thirst so it is honored.

| PRO TIP

Once you know what is needed for your lifestyle demands, set yourself up for success by making a visualization of the water that you won't be able to miss! We recommend setting water on the counter at the beginning of the day. That way you can actually see how much you've drunk and if you are meeting your base needs for the day.

If your kitchen counter is out of sight throughout the day, then find a bottle and figure out how many refills it's going to take to meet your daily intake.

Remember as we start this journey: don't get caught up in forced water intake. The visualization is to know where you are at present and if you are ignoring your thirst.

Curious about water weight? We retain fluid for a number of reasons, including excess sodium in the diet, hormonal imbalances, high levels of stress and inflammation. While you of course need to find and address the culprit behind consistent or excessive fluid retention with your doctor, you also need to drink up! Drinking water helps to flush stored water from the body. Often we retain fluid because we aren't taking in enough so the body wants to be sure it has water to utilize when needed.

CAROL + ALEX

| GIVE THANKS

"And whatever you do, in word or deed, do everything in the name of the Lord Jesus, giving thanks to God the Father through him." Colossians 3:17

Why are we beginning our soul habits with Give Thanks? By giving thanks to Him who provides perfectly designed nourishment for the exquisite body he knit together, you strengthen your "attitude of gratitude." It shifts your perspective from not having what you think you want to "what I have is more than enough." We know from studies that a life anchored by thankfulness is not only healthier, but more joy-filled than one that is not. We are built for praise. However, we are not just focused on worldly contentment and appreciation of its blessings. We are not focused on being happy because that feeling is purely circumstantial. The gratitude we refer to is far, far greater: God-centered gratitude. A gratitude that turns our gaze from the things or circumstances of this world to Jesus. Giving thanks, praising God, makes us aware of all we have been freely given: abundant provision, mercy, grace, forgiveness, the Holy Spirit, protection, strength, peace, and a love beyond measure. These gifts cannot be earned and therefore cannot be lost once received. Oh! How good is our God! He gives freely and steadfastly. Thanks be to God!!

> "Bless the LORD, everything he has created, everything in all his kingdom. Let all that I am bless the LORD." Psalm 103:22

Giving thanks is an act of recognition that only Jesus can satiate and fill the want. This week, practice giving thanks for the food you are about to eat. The healing that will come in your relationship with food through this simple act will be immeasurable. But, don't limit giving thanks to just food consumption! Throughout your day give thanks to your good, good Father. Thank him for your blessings and your lessons. Be grateful for when you do your best and when you are battling your brokenness. No matter your circumstance, remember you are covered by His grace. With Jesus, you have everything. What greater gift is there?

> "For I have learned in whatever situation I am to be content. I know how to be brought low. And I know how to abound. In any and every circumstance, I have learned the secret of facing plenty and hunger, abundance and need." Philippians 4:11-12

God-centered gratitude, transforms you from within because it is a life lived in humble awareness of His unfathomable grace. Choosing to give thanks for all things--in all circumstances--is a choice to stand in, under, and upon God and God's Truth alone. His grace is sufficient and it is your greatest blessing. Giving thanks will change you; it is the foundation of renewing your mind. Giving thanks for food (and your body) will be transformative; it will demolish the strongholds that keep you from a life honoring your body.

Enjoy this week (and we pray, the rest of your life) of inviting God into every interaction with food and for the gift of your body. We promise with God at the table (and as your mirror) you have taken the first steps to relationship with food and your body that will reap unimaginable fruit.

Choosing to live a grace-filled life and give thanks for all things is a choice to stand in, under, and upon God and God's Truth alone.

NOTES

AT THE KING'S TABLE

WATER RESTORES

Water Restores

> *"... He makes me lie down in green pastures, He leads me beside still waters, He restores my soul..."* Psalm 23:2–3a

> *"With joy you will draw water from the wells of salvation..."* Isaiah 12:3a

Water Strengthens

> *"And the Lord will guide you continually and satisfy your desire in scorched places and make your bones strong; and you shall be like a watered garden, like a spring of water, whose waters do not fail."* Isaiah 58:11

Water Makes New

> *"Let us draw near with a true heart in full assurance of faith, with our hearts sprinkled clean from an evil*

conscience and our bodies washed with pure water."
Hebrews 10:22

"Jesus answered, 'Truly, truly, I say to you, unless one
is born of water and the Spirit, he cannot enter the
kingdom of God." John 3:5

Water has always been symbolic of cleanliness and restoration. There's a reason baptisms aren't performed with oil or ash or some other substance. Water symbolizes cleaning off the old and being brought up in new life.

The human body is made up of approximately 55-60% water. It is an absolutely vital substance. Water is needed by the brain to produce hormones and neurotransmitters, it is needed in order to produce saliva and digestive fluids that break down food, it regulates core body temperature, it absorbs shock that protects the spinal cord, it delivers oxygen in the circulatory system, it is crucial to the filtration and detox system, it cushions joints, and is absolutely necessary for cells to function, grow, and reproduce. Metabolism is largely influenced by the micro process of cellular metabolism, or the sum total of chemical reactions that take place in the body in order to sustain life. Drinking enough water is step one to restoring your metabolism.

Refer back to Genesis 1. When God was creating existence as we know it, He chose to begin with water and earth. The earth would give rise to the plants that would feed the beasts, and both would become our life source. The water would be a vital life source for everything - earth, plants, beasts, and humans alike.

In short, water is essential. Why, then, have we gotten to a place where drinking this crucial life-supporting substance is so hard? A few reasons, but one being because our overstimulated palates prefer drinking fluids with more flavor. We've also settled into a hectic lifestyle that's always on-the-go, making having water on-hand difficult.

While it may not seem so significant, in a way, the culture we live in has distracted us from fully appreciating one of our Creator's first gifts to mankind. Chronic dehydration keeps us from reaching our healthiest state. We believe God wants us to live the life He's given us to the fullest. It's the little things, like drinking water, that add up to make the biggest difference.

| LEADER-LED DISCUSSION:

- This is a deeper look at the topic of drinking water. But like giving thanks, this seemingly mundane task is critical to transformation. Let's talk about water. Who loves to drink it? Who doesn't? Who is struggling with this habit? Who is recognizing their thirst and honoring it?

| FOOD IN ITS PLACE

> *"Therefore I tell you, do not be anxious about your life, what you will eat or what you will drink, nor about your body, what you will put on. Is life not more than food and the body more than clothing?"*
> *Matthew 6:25*

One of the unfortunate side effects of living in diet culture is finding your world suddenly revolves around food. Whether it's the fear of eating a specific food or the strong desire to eat that's being stifled by willpower and restriction, food rules your mind.

"Finally brothers and sisters, whatever is true, whatever is noble, whatever is right, whatever is pure, whatever is lovely, whatever is admirable – if that is excellent or praiseworthy – think about such things and the God of peace will be with you."
Philippians 4:8

"We demolish arguments and every pretension that sets itself up against the knowledge of God, and we take captive every thought and make it obedient to Christ." 2 Corinthians 10:5

God blessed us with minds that are extremely malleable. We can change the way our mind functions (and change actual structures) by taking thoughts captive and making them obedient to the example Christ set before us. Set your focus on things that are good - such as gratitude for food or a focus on the life that food allows you to live.

Chronic negative thinking also changes the way we think, but for the worse. Are obsessive or fearful thoughts about food productive? Do they result in peace or joy? Do they fuel vibrant physical and spiritual health? Or, do they enslave and imprison you in false guilt, shame, and various other strongholds?

Food was never meant to be what your life revolves around. Food provides the nourishment that supports life and the connection that builds community. It's something you traffic with at least 3 times a day, every day. It's important, you can't stop consuming it. But you can put it in its proper place: a life that does not worry about what you will eat or drink (Matthew 6:25-34).

| LEADER-LED DISCUSSION:

- Discuss the prevalence of food obsession or fears in the group.
- Discuss strategies to overcome these thoughts. What scriptures can you hold in your mind to defend against the negative thoughts?

| READING ASSIGNMENT

- Genesis 1:27
- Isaiah 26:3
- Isaiah 32:17
- Colossians 2:9-10
- Colossians 3:1-3

| ATTITUDE OF GRATITUDE

"Let them thank the Lord for His steadfast love, for His wondrous works to the children of man! For He satisfies the longing soul, and the hungry soul He fills with good things." Psalm 107:8-9

> "For everything created by God is good, and nothing is to be rejected if it is received with a heart of thanksgiving, for it is made holy by the word of God and prayer." 1 Timothy 4:4-5

When we embrace an attitude of true gratitude, we're stepping under the shelter of the Most High and will abide in the shadow of the Almighty (Psalm 91:1). By yielding to God and embracing His blessings as they fill our empty vessels, we're allowing His perfect love to cast out all fear. We're accepting that He is in fact in control, and just like the birds of the air, our needs will never be forgotten.

If only it were easy to be thankful for all things 100% of the time. We live in a culture that actively works to disconnect us from His provision. Diet culture has created a fear of food, mass confusion about what is "good" to eat, and a misguided focus on self image.

Untangling the confusion and re-learning what we all once knew so well is not easy. This is why we are beginning here, with gratitude. Putting on a heart of thanksgiving is like donning armor to protect against the weapons of culture that try to pull us further from what we know to be true. An attitude of true gratitude exposes the falsehoods of enemy strongholds. The intentionality of giving thanks empowers us to take every thought captive and make it obedient to Christ. It brings us back to the basics and lays a rock-solid foundation that will strengthen us on every battlefield.

| LEADER-LED DISCUSSION:

- Giving Thanks seems like a simple thing to do, yet the rush of everyday life can make even simple things difficult to follow through with. How easy or difficult has this habit been so far? Can you see this becoming a concrete habit in the future?
- How has this habit changed your attitude towards food so far?
- Open floor for questions and ending discussion; set time cap if necessary
- Set the next meeting day and time, if not already set.
- Conclude with prayer

| READING ASSIGNMENT

- John 10:10
- 2 Timothy 1:7

"Let them thank the Lord for His steadfast love, for His wondrous works to the children of man! For He satisfies the longing soul, and the hungry soul He fills with good things."

Psalm 107:8-9

WEEK 2
TRANSFORMATION
HABITS

FUEL YOUR BODY
EVERY SEED-BEARING PLANT
VEGETABLES & FRUIT
FEED YOUR SOUL
SPIRIT EMPOWERED FILLING THE WANT

"Then God said, I give you every seed-bearing plant on the face of the whole earth and every tree that has fruit with seed in it. They will be yours for food." Genesis 1:29

| HABIT CHECK!

The habits and mindset you have developed around food have been practiced for many years. Week one brings your current habits to the surface, allowing for a renewed awareness in the areas that need Spirit conviction. Throughout this six weeks, make sure you continue to practice each habit introduced. We have intentionally introduced habits to logically build upon each other. Proper hydration is key to keeping your digestive system happy and moving things. Give thanks will be reinforced as you marvel this week at the diverse beauty of God's abundant provision. If you feel overwhelmed or any habit slipping, stop, breathe, and pray. Or, as we like to say: SLOW YOUR ROLL and take it to the Cross. Take all the time you need and remember to show yourself grace throughout this journey.

EVERY SEED-BEARING PLANT: VEGETABLES & FRUIT

Eat your vegetables! How many of you heard this simple phrase repeatedly during your childhood? How many of you now repeat this mantra as a parent? Well, buckle up, because this week's Fuel Habit: EAT YOUR VEGETABLES & FRUIT!

The first question to ask: why should the foundation and bulk of your food intake be vegetables and fruit? The nutrition science answer: fresh produce is packed with micronutrients and fiber. It is perfectly designed (thank you Lord for your perfect care) to nourish your body. When you eat sufficient vegetables and fruit your hunger cues become trustworthy, cravings diminish, mental clarity increases, and your energy levels stabilize. The proper intake of produce, as well, lowers the risk of many diseases. The God rooted answer as to why vegetables and fruit should be the foundation and bulk of your food intake comes from, well, the Bible. The first Biblical mention of food occurs in Genesis 1:29:

> "Then God said, "Look! I have given you every seed-bearing plant throughout the earth and all the fruit trees for your food."

When seeking the truth about your body, doesn't it make sense to ask its Creator? God begins with vegetables and fruit. So... is it any surprise that your body functions best when the foundation and bulk of your intake is...drum roll: vegetables and fruit. The fruit of the Spirit comes when we first seek our all-knowing God. Take a moment and give thanks to God for the beauty and simplicity of his perfect plan for your body.

NEWS FLASH: YOUR BODY DOES NOT RESPOND TO CALORIES. IT RESPONDS TO NUTRIENTS.

Even diet culture cannot completely disregard God's perfect plan. All diets and their cleverly renamed lifestyles agree on one thing: vegetables and fruit are the foundation of health. Diet culture accepts that produce, because of its nutrient density and fiber content, helps you naturally control your caloric intake (more on this in a bit). A nourished body is satiated and, therefore, you are less likely to overeat, overindulge, or succumb to cravings. Without a solid foundation of vegetables and fruit, your body will be nutrient deprived. You will simply be locked in a never-ending battle with hunger and cravings. Where diet culture's interest in produce is limited to controlling your caloric intake, we want you to understand that all this science points back to God's truth. The Creator of your body intelligently designed its provision. He began with vegetables and fruit and lo' and behold you function best when you follow suit. God's provision not only physically equips you to fulfill your kingdom purpose; it quiets your body so you can focus on the provider and not the provision. Vegetables and fruit are part of God's simple yet perfect plan to free you from being enslaved to appetite.

Restriction based diets ignore the intelligent design of your body. A body well-fueled is a body that knows when enough is enough.

Rather than a diet mindset of restriction and elimination (yes, the more corrosive ones even demonize certain vegetables and fruit, making us fearful of potatoes and bananas), we begin by seeking God's truth. We trust that He knows what we need. Our bodies need "every seed-bearing plant….and all the fruit trees for food." Honor your body and humbly submit to His truth. Fill your body's need, and you will battle the desires of your flesh far less. Nourish your body as God intended and you will experience the fruit of the Spirit: self-control and peace. Fill yourself with vegetables and fruit to nourish it, to build a sustainable relationship with food where it is not the focus of your thoughts, and to once and for all free yourself from the stronghold of dieting.

All diets--and because we cannot repeat it enough: their cleverly renamed lifestyles-- restrict calories through different means. Their various methods of restriction and elimination do, in truth, produce quick weight-loss results. However, the results are always temporary (98.2% of the time) because the only weapon in your dieting arsenal is willpower. Diets ignore YOU. They ignore and dismiss God's truth. They ignore your brokenness (we would argue they feed off it) and, at some point, your willpower will falter or your circumstance will interrupt. Hence, the temporary results for the vast majority of dieters. If you need to lose weight, can we tell you calories don't matter? Unfortunately, as much as we would like to say they don't, calories cannot be completely ignored. We have a finely tuned net energy balance. Over consumption will lead to weight gain. However, if you honor your body according to God's plan detailed in the first book, first chapter of the Bible--fueling it, first and most abundantly, with nutrient dense vegetables and fruit--over consumption of calories will be far less likely. Rather than dieting (restricting and eliminating), have you tried adding all that your body was designed to need? We can say with absolute confidence: you can trust God. Remember, he not only doesn't want you enslaved to your appetite, He wants you not to worry about food. Surrender to His Truth.

Embrace the greatest weapon in your transformation arsenal: God's Truth.

| HOW MUCH IS ENOUGH?

Our intention each week when we address "how much" is never rooted in restriction. Rather, "how much" is always focused on getting enough. Through awareness you discover what you need to best fuel your body. The goal is always to honor your body so that it no longer battles you but supports the demands of your life. The goal is to demolish diet culture strongholds. Sufficient intake of produce will free you from several. The optimal goal for vegetables and fruit for adults is 7-11 servings per day (the baseline 5-7). However, be cautious, we don't want to reinforce the diet stronghold of measuring. The truth, most of us do not consume near enough vegetables and fruit. We need to eat more! Please don't restrict or measure vegetables or fruit in any way! The beautiful outcome of a well-nourished body: it allows you to reconnect and trust your hunger cues. Over time a body that works for you will balance your consumption to support your net energy balance. All this to say: we do not want anyone wasting one precious moment of their God-purposed life measuring carrots or worrying about which, or how much, fruit. Just make sure you are eating enough!

A simple visual to make sure you are consuming sufficient vegetables and fruit each day as you work towards the optimal amount that your body and lifestyle requires:

1 serving equals:

Non-starchy and leafy vegetables: open hand or half your plate at each meal
Starchy vegetables and fruit: cupped palm or quarter of your plate

Example for OPTIMAL daily intake:

2 servings at Breakfast: Eggs with sauteed greens and tomatoes; or a Smoothie with greens and fruit; or yogurt with fresh fruit

4 servings at Lunch: plate or bowl filled with leafy greens, add chopped veggies and fruit (with added protein source); leafy greens and chopped veggies on your sandwich with fruit

3-4 servings at Dinner: half your plate with roasted veggies, a potato, and a side salad with whatever protein

Total possible in just three meals: 9-10 servings

| PRO-TIPS:

Eat a diverse VARIETY of vegetables and fruit (all the colors) to ensure complete nutrient intake.

Making seasonal selections helps connect to God's plan as different vegetables and fruit thrive in different seasons, each designed to provide the energy and nutrients we need for that season as well as comfort (more energy and cooling in the longer days of summer; more filling and warmth in the dark, cold days of winter).

If you discover you don't eat much in the way of vegetables and fruit, then please increase your intake slowly. Respect the increased fiber and give your digestive system a hot minute to catch up.

Start in the grocery store: If half your cart is vegetables and fruit, then you are more likely to have vegetables and fruit become half your daily consumption.

Throwing away too much produce? Stock up on frozen and canned vegetables (watch added sodium or sugars in canned). Don't destroy the good for the perfect!   Canned vegetables are better than no vegetables and frozen produce is perfect for smoothies, baking, quick prep, and always having it on hand. As well, frozen and canned vegetables are already chopped (less work in the kitchen). Remember: If your vegetable and fruit drawer is a pre-compost staging area, you will not develop healthy consumption of vegetables and fruit. Rotten vegetables and fruit do not encourage a mindset of "ooh! I want to keep purchasing and eating more of this!"

Caution on canned or jarred fruit: added sugars and syrup are common, increasing empty calorie consumption. Frozen fruit is fabulous in every way!

A thought on juice and juicing: Juicing, whether vegetables or fruit, removes the fiber (and, in our humble opinion the joy of the crunch!). Fiber is so necessary and so neglected in our diets:

- it slows down the energy release from carbohydrates, allowing your body to efficiently use it rather than storing the excess
- it creates fullness to naturally control over-consumption.

PS. Blending is not the same as juicing...fiber is broken down, but it does remain.

Love Note: This habit is about getting enough vegetables and fruit. Please don't allow the world and its gurus cause you to worry if you are eating too much. As we move through these six weeks and you give this area of your life over to God, your relationship with food will bear fruit!

CAROL + ALEX

"For everything there is a season...."

SEASONAL PRODUCE

WINTER

Apples
Arugula ·
Asian Pears
Blood Oranges
Brussel Sprouts
Cabbage
Carrots
Celery
Chayote Squash
Citrons
Clementines
Collards
Escarole
Fennel
Guava
Jicama
Kale
Kumquats

Meyer Lemons
Mustard Greens
Olives
Parsnips
Persimmon
Pomelos
Potatoes
Pumpkins
Oranges
Radicchio
Radishes (varieties)
Sage
Star Fruit
Swiss Chard
Tangerines
Turnips
Winter Squash
Yams

SPRING

Apricots
Artichokes
Arugula
Asparagus
Avocado
Bananas
Bok Choy
Broccoli

Broccoli rabe
Cabbage
Carrots
Celeriac
Celery
Cherries
Collard Greens
Cress

Endive
Fennel
Garlic
Greens (Cooking)
Guava
Kale
Lettuce
Limes
Mushrooms
Onions
Pea Shoots
Peas
Pineapple
Potatoes
Radishes

Rhubarb
Romanesco
Scallions
Snow peas
Sorrel
Spinach
Spring Baby Lettuce
Sprouts
Strawberries
Sugar Snap Peas
Sweet Corn
Swiss Chard
Vidalia Onions
Watercress

SUMMER

Apples
Apricots
Arugula
Avocado
Bananas
Beets
Bell Peppers
Blackberries
Blueberries
Bok Choy
Boysenberries
Burdock
Carrots
Cantaloupe
Casaba Melon
Celery

Cherries
Chile Peppers
Collard Greens
Corn
Cress
Cucumbers
Endive
Eggplant
Fennel
Figs
Garlic
Grapefruit
Grapes
Green Beans
Green Peas
Honeydew Melon

Kiwi
Lima Beans
Mangos
Nectarines
Okra
Onions
Peaches
Plums
Raspberries
Romanesco
Scallions

Shallots
Shelling beans
Sprouts
Strawberries
Summer Squash
Tomatillos
Tomatoes
Watermelon
Zucchini

FALL

Acorn Squash
Apples
Arugula
Avocado
Bananas
Beets
Bell Peppers
Bok Choy
Broccoli
Broccoli rabe
Brussel Sprouts
Burdock
Cabbage
Carrots
Cauliflower
Celeriac
Celery
Chayote Squash
Cherimoya
Coconuts

Collard Greens
Cranberries
Cress
Dates
Diakon Radish
Endive
Fennel
Figs
Garlic
Ginger
Grapes
Greens (cooking)
Green Beans
Jicama
Kale
Lettuces
Limes
Mangos
Melon
Mushrooms

Onions

Parsnips

Peas

Pears

Pineapple

Pomegranate

Potatoes

Pumpkin

Radishes

Raspberries

Romanesco

Rutabagas

Scallions

Shelling beans

Spinach

Sprouts

Sweet Potatoes

Swiss Chard

Turnips

Winter Squash

Yams

| SPIRIT EMPOWERMENT: FILLING THE WANT

"Come to me all you who are weary and burdened, and I will give you rest." Matthew 11:28

The second soul habit embraces the tension between our flesh and our spirit. Desires and emotions are integral to who we were made to be. Without them we would not be hardwired to desperately need and desire a relationship with God, nor would we be unable to love as we are commanded to love. However, we live in a fallen world, wrapped in the brokenness of our flesh. Praise Jesus for his surrender. Through His obedience we received the Holy Spirit. The Holy Spirit protects and leads us to our promised Kingdom wholeness. With the Spirit, surrendered to God's will, our desires and emotions are tempered with self-control, patience, moderation, kindness and are redirected to all that is true, noble, right, and pure. We are called to put our flesh second to our spirit so that our lives--in everything we do--glorify God. Praise God that his love is perfect and his grace sufficient. God did not leave us to battle our worldly brokenness alone and He covered it through Christ.

Our relationship with food is rife with tension. We keenly feel the struggle between our flesh (desires/emotions) and our spirit (self-control) in this relationship. Food is a necessity, but it also creates SO MANY EMOTIONS! Food is a source of celebration, happiness, and provides comfort. Equally, diet culture has caused food to become a source of anxiety, false guilt, and shame. By its very nature, our relationship with food in a culture that has an abundance is emotional. It is not a surprise that all of our clients tell us they struggle with "emotional eating." The answer is not to conquer (or ignore) your emotions. Emotions are a God-given gift. Rather, we must learn to not be led by our emotions. We are called to seek God above how we feel or what we desire in the moment. In other words: we are called to set our spirit above our flesh so that we are not ruled by, or fall prey to, fleshly desires and emotions. Willpower protects in the moment, allowing you to seek God. The Holy Spirit empowers your Christ-mindedness.

I Want. He Fills.

Adding to the emotional relationship we have with food are entrenched, rote behaviors (you come home sad or scuffed up from school: a treat will make it better; eat all your vegetables or no dessert, etc.). The first step to unpack our complex relationship with food is to identify your emotional triggers and entrenched behaviors. You must gain full awareness of both in order to grow mindful of the thoughts or circumstances that lead to mindless food consumption (eating when not hungry), over-consumption (eating beyond the point of full), and even willful refusal to eat when hungry or food fears created by diet culture. There are clearly too many triggers to list, but those we most commonly hear are:

Exhaustion
Boredom
Disappointment
Sadness
Anxiety
Guilt
Social situations (food set out at work, celebrations, gatherings, arguments with others)

No doubt, you can think of many others. Our triggers and entrenched behaviors are as unique as we are. The key to honing your Spirit led self-control over your flesh is to become mindful of your specific triggers and behaviors then take them to the Cross. Through habitual reactions and behaviors, food has become overly associated with, and controlled by, our emotions or situation (our flesh and the world). Food is not the problem. Unfortunately, it is also not the solution: only Jesus. Take note of when you mindlessly eat, overeat, or skip eating. What were you feeling and/or what happened in the moments or time before? What is the situation you find yourself in when you mindlessly eat, overeat, or refuse to eat when needed? Strive to separate food consumption from the trigger, the behavior, the situation, or diet culture fear. Once these are identified--when your flesh and the world gets the better of your spirit--the next step is to bring every bit of it--all of you--to the Cross. Yield all to His will and open your heart to discern His. At the foot of the Cross is where healing, rest, discernment, and wisdom are found. Through the Word, prayer, and being fully surrendered to God is how you are strengthened (and healed) against the tension raging within and around you. Trust us, because we are broken messes as well, when we tell you that the enemy will use your flesh and the world to take possession of your mind. The enemy seeks to draw you far from the shelter of God. What a blessing that you can bring every bit of you and your circumstance to the foot of the Cross. You will marvel at the peace and clarity that will occur. God gave you His Spirit to redirect your thoughts, calm your desires and emotions, and fill your want; it is through His grace alone that we overcome our flesh. It is through His grace alone that we are able to put down our struggle with food.

> "Now to Him who is able to do immeasurably more than all we ask or imagine. According to His power that is at work with us. To Him be glory in the church and in Christ Jesus throughout all generations, forever and ever!" Ephesians 3:20

Trust this eternal truth: we have a good, good Father. It is impossible for Him to be anything but good--it is His innate nature. He is the Good Shepherd who walks with us through all circumstances. He is the Creator and the Redeemer; He created all and restores all. He is perfect in every way; His mercies never fail, and His grace is sufficient. His love for you, knowing the tension you live in between flesh and spirit, in between worldly brokenness and Kingdom wholeness, gifted you not only with Jesus's sacrifice but His indwelling Spirit. God knows when you are empty and at your weakest, His power is able to be made perfect in you. Through His grace, Jesus's sacrifice, and the gift of the Holy Spirit you are a vessel designed to overflow so that you plant seeds and shine His light to the world. Empty yourself of self, of the world, cling to the Cross so that His Spirit fills you to the point of overflowing.

Trust that he wants so much more for you than constant struggle with food:

> "But don't be so concerned about perishable things like food. Spend your energy seeking the eternal life that the Son of Man can give you. For God the Father has given me the seal of his approval." John 6:27

NOTES

AT THE KING'S TABLE

YOURS FOR FOOD

"Then God said, I give you every seed-bearing plant on the face of the whole earth and every tree that has fruit with seed in it. They will be yours for food."
Genesis 1:29

Your mother was right - EAT YOUR VEGGIES! The vegetables and fruit that God created are perfectly designed to provide you with the nourishment needed to lead a healthy and kingdom purposed life. The same God who authored the story of all that has passed and all that will come is the One who created you. He created you in His own image, intentionally purposed. And central to our purpose is the experience of the joy of Christ and to fill the world with His truth.

Do you trust that God has given you all you need to live out your purpose? Even things as simple and mundane as the vegetables and fruit needed to fuel your health so that you are physically equipped to fulfill His purpose?

He goes before you. He prepares a table for you to meet all of your physical and spiritual needs. Your table overflows with the abundance of His provision. It includes everything your body will ever need.

Today we challenge you to shift your perspective from "I have to eat [xyz]" to "I get to enjoy the nourishment my Creator has provided for me." This mindset shift goes hand-in-hand with your first Feed Your Soul Habit, Giving Thanks.

We are, after all, pretty lucky to have a Father who sees that our every last need is provided for.

| LEADER-LED DISCUSSION:

- Open discussion about eating veggies and fruit. Is this hard for the group? Easy? Discuss how diet culture has created fear around certain vegetables and fruit.
- Discuss the truth we find in Genesis and the significance of God's wisdom about what our bodies truly need. Discuss why His plan is good.
- Share storage and prep tips as well as recipes. Sharpen each other.
- Does shifting your perspective from "have to" to "get to" help with eating more vegetables and fruit? Why or why not?

| LET NOT YOUR HEARTS BE TROUBLED

"Let not your hearts be troubled. Believe in God; believe also in me. In my Father's house are many rooms. If it were not so, would I have told you that I go to prepare a place for you? And if I go and prepare a place for you, I will come again and will take you to myself, that where I am you may be also. And you know the way to where I am going." Thomas said to him, "Lord, we do not know where you are going. How can we know the way?" Jesus said to him, "I am the way, and the truth, and the life. No one comes to the Father except through me. If you had known me, you would have known my Father also. From now on you do know him and have seen him." John 14:1-7

We are a stressed out nation. Incidences of emotional and mental imbalances and disorders are rising at an alarming rate. There's a lot that we can blame for this: social media, fast-paced lifestyles, and all of the other consequences of being alive in the modern day. But there's One (and only one) that can take our stress away and fill us with peace.

The Prince of Peace came so that we might come to know the love of the Father. Christ accepted unthinkable suffering so that we might have life, and have it to the fullest. The next time you find stress or anxiety interfering with your life, stop and know that He is God. He will fight your battles for you, you must only be still. There is room in the Father's house - Christ himself has prepared a place for you.

"I will not leave you as orphans; I will come to you. Yet a little while and the world will see me no more, but you will see me. Because I live, you also will live. In that day you will know that

I am in my Father, and you in me, and I in you. Whoever has my commandments and keeps them, he it is who loves me. And he who loves me will be loved by my Father, and I will love him and manifest myself to him." Judas (not Iscariot) said to him, "Lord, how is it that you will manifest yourself to us, and not to the world?" Jesus answered him, "If anyone loves me, he will keep my word, and my

Father will love him, and we will come to him and make our home with him. Whoever does not love me does not keep my words. And the word that you hear is not mine but the Father's who sent me." John 14:18-24

Many of the stressors we face are intertwined with fear and anxiety in some way - either fear causes the stress or comes as a result of the stress. Fear cannot exist in the presence of perfect love. In times of stress (and times of peace), hold tight to the Truth and fill your mind with the Word of God. Here you will find rest. In Him you will find safety and comfort.

Make your home in the Lord by dwelling in His word.

> *"These things I have spoken to you while I am still with you. But the Helper, the Holy Spirit, whom the Father will send in my name, he will teach you all things and bring to your remembrance all that I have said to you. Peace I leave with you; my peace I give to you. Not as the world gives do I give to you. Let not your hearts be troubled, neither let them be afraid. You heard me say to you, 'I am going away, and I will come to you.' If you loved me, you would have rejoiced, because I am going to the Father, for the Father is greater than I. And now I have told you before it takes place, so that when it does take place you may believe.*
>
> *I will no longer talk much with you, for the ruler of this world is coming. He has no claim on me, but I do as the Father has commanded me, so that the world may know that I love the Father. Rise, let us go from here." John 14:25-31*

The Helper, the Holy Spirit, which is sent by God in the name of Jesus, will be your teacher. Lean fully on the wisdom of the Father and the Spirit that resides within you to navigate the stress and anxiety of today's lifestyle. Stress doesn't just erode your physical health, it can work to separate you from your Father. Or, you can choose to use stressful situations to lean into God and watch the Prince of Peace direct you in all that you do.

| LEADER-LED DISCUSSION:

- Open discussion about the topic of stress and anxiety. In what ways do these two things affect the group?
- How often do you think to look to God in stressful situations?
- What Bible verses can you hold in your mind to anchor you in the Truth when things go awry? Think outside the verses outlined today; allow the group to contribute their favorite verses.

| READING ASSIGNMENT

- 2 Timothy 2:4
- Psalm 51:10

| OH! OH! OH!

Willpower is a finite resource.

To truly transform, not the superficial Tuesday Transformation of diet culture, but a transformation that renews your mind, you must make a clear distinction between a worldly view and a God-centered life. Diet culture worldly view anchors your success and failure to the finite resource willpower. Willpower is self-reliant and therefore is God designed to falter. It is a gift--a momentary hard stop-

-to protect us from temptation. A breath. A chance to turn your attention from the desire to God. God calls you to rely on Him and to anchor yourself in His truth. He is your help and firm foundation. He is your infinite resource to resist temptation.

In "Desiring God," John Piper quotes David Smith, "When it comes to living a successful Christian life, and resisting the power of temptation, simply saying 'No! No! No!' won't suffice. We must learn to say 'Oh! Oh! Oh!'" Piper continues, "In other words, being amazed at God is essential to fighting sin."

Can we get an Amen!!

God's word is clear. Eating to excess, gluttony, is sin (note: overweight and obesity are not sin; a person might be overweight and/or obese without eating to excess/ gluttony). Gluttony is allowing your appetite to master and enslave you. It is allowing your desire for food to supplant your desire for God.

> "Their destiny is destruction, their god is their stomach, and their glory is in their shame. Their mind is set on earthly things." Philippians 3:19

> "And put a knife to your throat if you are given to gluttony." Proverbs 23:2

The worldly view, or diet culture mindset, tells us to rely on willpower, to simply say "No! No! No!" However, at its best, willpower is merely a kickstart in the fight against gluttony. In his book, *Willpower*, social psychologist Roy Baumeister concludes that human beings possess a finite supply of willpower.

He compares willpower to muscle. Muscles enable us to begin and do work for a period of time. However, like muscle strength, willpower rapidly depletes as it is used. Simply saying "No!" to food cravings and fleshly desires is a short-sighted strategy. God gifted you the willpower to begin the battle against temptation and to choose right habits. However, believing that willpower is sufficient is folly; it is an enemy stronghold. At its core, the belief that we possess unlimited willpower in the battle against temptation is self worship (Numbers 11:18-20).

Diet culture mindset's reliance on willpower ignores "Oh! Oh! Oh!"

| LEADER-LED DISCUSSION:

- How many times have you relied on willpower and "No! No! No!" to reach a desired weight or health goal?
- Did willpower prove sufficient?
- How has diet culture mindset imprisoned you (false guilt, shame, avoidance of social settings, judgement of others, robbed you of time from God, from loved ones)

| A DIFFERENT WAY

Do ALL things for the glory of God. Self-control, Biblically speaking, comes through the power of the Holy Spirit. Living a God-centered, Kingdom seeking life is reliant on the indwelling Holy Spirit to guard us against sin. Why? Because God is the restorer. His love, grace, and mercy transform. Unlike the finite strength of willpower, the power and strength of God is without limitation. How do we tap into His supernatural power to resist temptation? We put God before us. We place God's Truth as the foundation, center and end goal of our lives.

> "You were taught, with regard to your former way of life, to put off your old self, which is being corrupted by its deceitful desires; to be made

new in the attitude of your minds; and to put on the new self, created to be like God in true righteousness and holiness." Ephesians 4:22-23

Putting God before us recognizes that moderation and self-control do not earn God's favor. Rather, God's relentless love, forgiveness, and gift of the Holy Spirit motivate us to walk a narrow path. God's grace is sufficient. When we fully submit to His ways, everything changes. His grace makes a life of moderation and self-control joy-filled because through it we honor Him.

How do we put God before ourselves? By actively pursuing an intimate relationship with Him through our praise, worship, prayer and focused time spent in His Word. God transforms our mindset when we seek Him first in ALL things, especially in areas of weakness. Remember He fills our want. He is our strength, a strength that can never be depleted.

"But he said to me, "My grace is sufficient for you, for my power is made perfect in weakness." Therefore I will boast all the more gladly of my weaknesses, so that the power of Christ may rest upon me." 2 Cor 12:9

| **LEADER-LED DISCUSSION:**

- Do you trust God fully in this life struggle or do you fall prey to diet gurus and trends?
- In our relationship with food, how can you put God first to guard you against overindulgence and live in "Oh! Oh! Oh!"?
- How is God-inspired moderation and self-control different from willpower?

| HONORING THE BODY HONORS GOD

As we have learned, the pursuit of diet culture mindset, the path of perfection, is not one of moderation. Its path is as ruinous to our physical and emotional health as is gluttony because it is anchored in a worldly view: it looks to our own power rather than trusting God's. God calls us to resist ALL temptation through relationship with Him.

A life guided by moderation and self-control is not an imprisoned life; it is a humbly obedient life. It recognizes that we NEED God. It is worth repeating that we don't practice restraint to master ourselves. Rather we walk a narrow path to bring glory to God and to be able to fulfill His purpose for our lives. Chronic dieting and gluttony drain our emotional and physical well-being. Both pull us from God's protection. Both deny the truth that our body does not belong to us.

> "Do you not know that your bodies are temples of the Holy Spirit, who is in you, whom you have received from God? You are not your own; you were bought at a price. Therefore honor God with your bodies." 1 Cor 6:19-20

As with all of His creation, our bodies belong to God and He calls us to be good stewards. As believers, our body is now a sacred space for the Holy Spirit. A temple bought with the precious blood of Jesus. Our culture of deprivation and overindulgence has damaged our health: we are a people unable to rest, riddled with disease and chronic illnesses and rife with hormonal imbalances that wreak havoc on our emotions and mental clarity. Sadly, our current state of dis-ease limits our ability to fully fulfill God's purpose for our lives.

| LEADER-LED DISCUSSION:

- How well are you currently honoring your body by feeding it God's bounty? Where are areas you can improve (vegetables, fresh fruit, protein, whole grains, legumes, healthy fats)?

- When you choose to indulge, what are ways you protect yourself from overindulging? (Recognizing foods, situations or emotions that trigger you; creating boundaries to keep indulgence in its proper amount; being aware of thoughts such as "I've earned this" "I messed up and was bad" "I am so mad at myself for eating....").

- Are your protective measures to practice moderation, self-control, and restraint healthy or do you tend to fall into a fear-based relationship with food? (All or nothing attitude; diet culture mindset)

- How often do you recognize that you were created in God's image and honor the gift of your body: all it does for you and all it is capable of? Do you thank God for your body or are you trapped in worldly thoughts that diminish your beauty?

| CONCLUSION

This week's feed your soul habit is asking us to make perhaps the most difficult distinction when it comes to our well being. Looking to the world, we will continue to bounce back and forth between "given to appetite" and a self-loathing/vanity that drives over restriction. We will continue to be failed by the finite resource of willpower because it fuels hubris.

When we seek God's way, we can begin to recognize the difference between hunger (the body needs nourishment) and appetite (fleshly desire/temptation/cravings/ boredom/emotional). Living a life of restraint, one anchored in God's Truth frees us from the prison of diet culture mindset. Let's fix our eyes on God in this area of our life.

Remember:

- God desires nothing but our good.
- His ways are true.
- Being obedient to a life of moderation and self-control honors God's grace; it is joy-filled.

This week's habit, when anchored in "Oh! Oh! Oh!", is transformative.

| LEADER-LED DISCUSSION:

- Open the floor for questions; set time cap if necessary
- Set next meeting time, if not already set
- Conclude with prayer

| READING ASSIGNMENT

- Romans 13:14
- Colossians 3:17
- Proverbs 25:27
- Psalm 34:5

"Then God said, I give you every seed-bearing plant on the face of the whole earth and every tree that has fruit with seed in it. They will be yours for food."

Genesis 1:29

WEEK 3
TRANSFORMATION
HABITS

FUEL YOUR BODY
Recognizing Fullness
FEED YOUR SOUL
In All Your Ways

Habit Check!

We pray you are beginning to reap rewards of a shifted mindset: from elimination and restriction to adding all that is good. A body that is well-hydrated and well-nourished works for you. Honoring what your body needs, rather than falling prey to willful restriction and fear-filled eliminations, is empowering and freeing. Keep drinking your water and eating your vegetables and fruit! Give thanks to God for creating you in His image. You are wonderfully and fearfully made. Give thanks for His abundant provision and wisdom in its care. As your "new self" habits strengthen, allowing you to trust (and dare we say appreciate) your body, and you shift from faith in diets to Jesus, we pray you are beginning to experience the fruit of the Spirit!

| RECOGNIZING FULLNESS

"The temptations in your life are no different from what others experience. And God is faithful. He will not allow the temptation to be more than you can stand. When you are tempted, he will show you a way out so that you can endure." 1 Corinthians 10:13

The Okinawans teach their children "hara hachi bu." It means: eat only until you are 80% full. Our prayer is that we begin to teach our children (and ourselves) the same.

We, as a culture, have been disconnected from our innate ability to sense when we are full. Today, most of us eat to the point of stuffed. We simply miss the cues from our body. Eating to over-full results in the consumption of excess of calories, which leads to unwanted weight gain and gastric distress. Consistent over-eating can raise our lipid levels, increase our risk for Type 2 diabetes, and contribute to a host of hormonal imbalances.

Why do we overeat? Overeating is fueled by many things:

food products lacking nutrients, stress, oversized portions at restaurants, lack of sleep, insufficient balance of macronutrients, massive food availability from industrialized growing practices, hyper- palatable foods, lack of food variety causing diminished satisfaction, in search of comfort, and rushed or distracted eating to name just a few. In addition, the reasons behind overeating—and the consistent habit of overeating— have confused and silenced the cues our bodies are designed to send. We mistake thirst for hunger and do not hear our stomach's yellow warning light. Our brain is about 20 minutes behind our stomach. When the hesitant thought "should I take another bite" occurs, that is the stomach shouting: "I am full."

Recognizing fullness isn't something to do; rather, it is mindfulness, an intention.

Sustainable health and transforming your relationship with food is built on a two-part foundation: what we do and what we think. The two are inextricably and beautifully intertwined. What we DO makes us more thoughtful; what we think about and on becomes what we do. We have already had you address some of the reasons behind overeating in our habits to date:

1. Sufficient Hydration makes clear the difference between thirst and hunger cues.
2. Giving Thanks reduces our stress, provides comfort, and diminishes the likelihood of rushing and distraction while consuming food.
3. Vegetables and Fruit provide the nutrient density that signals your body to release fullness hormones as well as restoring your palate to become sensitive to hyper-palatable foods.
4. Spirit Empowerment: filling the want: brings awareness to emotional triggers, giving us a moment to run to yielded faith rather than be mindlessly imprisoned by the desires of our flesh and the stronghold of willpower.

This week we want to deepen your mindful roots in this area of your relationship with food. When you eat, sit. Truly. Remove distractions (cell phones, TV, etc.). Bow your head and give thanks. Chew your food slowly and thoroughly (much like with eat your veggies, mom was right when she chided you to chew your food a hundred times). Chewing thoroughly slows down eating. It enables proper absorption of nutrients, gives you time to know when you are full, and reduces the likelihood of eating to overfull. Make sure your plate has plenty of fresh vegetables or fruit to nourish your body and provide the filling benefits of fiber. Listen for your internal cue that you have had your fill. Honor it. Don't take that additional bite. Give your brain a chance to catch up, and then enjoy feeling satisfied rather than stuffed. Return to old-fashioned table etiquette. Proper table etiquette often required putting down your utensil between each bite, allowing not only time to chew slowly and thoroughly, but also opening the opportunity for fellowship with those gathered around your table. Learn to appreciate the value of food (how it nourishes and honors your body) rather than obsessing over food (let go of negative food/diet language and practices). Enjoy eating! What?! Yes, food is a blessing and was intended for our sustenance and PLEASURE (God didn't *have to* give us taste buds or make food look and smell so wonderful). It is heartbreaking how diet culture has made food become such a source of shame, worry, and anxiety. Negative food/diet language and practices have caused us to rush through eating, to eat in isolation,or to skip eating. Eating has become a joyless chore. Worse, often when we eat false guilt is triggered and we feel the heavy burden of shame.

Eating IS NOT a guilty pleasure; it doesn't need to be rushed, hidden, or skipped.

As you can see, we've laid most of the groundwork for this fuel your body habit. Hopefully, recognizing fullness is becoming easier and soon it will be something you are doing without even trying! However, at present you may still be woefully disconnected from recognizing fullness due to years of sowing seeds in the world of restriction/binge diet culture. In addition to building new habits and learning to enjoy eating, please be mindful when you overeat to learn. Ask Why? What were the triggers or practices? How did you feel after overeating? Was there a moment where you ignored a signal? In other words, be aware without sitting in judgement. Show yourself some grace. Recognizing fullness takes practice and healing!

Recognizing fullness
is another brick laid
securely in the narrow
path of self-control
and moderation.

| REFLECTION

Fullness is JUST satisfied; not stuffed. That next bite is possible, even desired. No doubt, you have many experiences that you took the next bite and then immediately felt remorse because you became physically uncomfortable. Learn from your past experiences so that you give your brain a chance to hear your stomach.

In other words, fullness is not a **quantifiable amount**. Rather, it is a **conscious effort** to not overeat; it is an intentional choice to be mindful of, and reconnect to, your body's God-given signals. It is a disciplined habit to know when to leave your meal, so in several minutes you feel satisfied rather than stuffed. When you choose to eat slowly and become mindful of your appetite, even when you are feeding your soul, you will not overeat. Appetite awareness will serve you well....lest you vomit.

| IN ALL YOUR WAYS

"Trust in the Lord with all your heart, and do not lean on your own understanding. In all your ways, acknowledge him, and he will make your paths straight." Proverbs 3:5-6

If you're familiar with scripture, then you've probably heard the verse written above. Like the 23rd Psalm, it's one of those verses that is printed on bookmarks, embroidered on quilts, and memorized in vacation Bible school. Trust in the Lord with all of your heart. Don't lean on your own understanding. Acknowledge Him. He will make your paths straight.

Unfortunately, it's also one of the verses that's often used as a spiritual band-aid, a quick mantra repeated in times of distress to provide immediate relief. When a verse is taken out of its intended context and used as a band-aid, its value and weight are reduced significantly. Verses like these, while pleasant to the ears, can also provide invaluable instruction on how to carry out life.

So what is this verse saying? First, it's saying to place your trust in the Lord. In an excellent sermon entitled *Trusting the Trustworthy One*, the pastor explained that who or what you trust is who or what you worship. And who or what you worship, is who or what you become like.

Out of context, this verse is often used to remind you that God is almighty and sovereign, and when things start to turn upside down He can be trusted to make all things work for the good of those who love Him.

Is this true? Without a doubt it is. But is this what this verse is getting at? Not entirely. The first instruction in this verse is to place all of your trust in the Lord always, to worship Him with your life so that you can become like Him through your walk with Christ. If you trust that the Lord is who He says He is, you'll live out your every day worshiping Him and mirroring His heart. There's a lot more depth in it when looked at through that perspective. He's not just a lifevest; He controls the waves and can give you the power to walk on water.

Onto the second piece of instruction: "And lean not on your own understanding." This line can be used as a band-aid when life's situations spin out of your "control," or it can be a reminder to live your everyday life with the Truth and the Trinity as your support. When you lean on something, you place your weight on it to support you. Now you only see in part, but He sees in full. Let His wisdom be what supports you. Be a yielded vessel to what He is trying to tell you and don't let your own head get in the way.

The next line of instruction: "In all your ways acknowledge Him..." To know--in Biblical context--is to have a deep understanding of something through an involved experience. To acknowledge God in all of your ways is to know God as the God of your [*insert anything here*], and to deepen your relationship with Him in every area of life. He is the God of your relationships, the God of your finances, the God of your career, etc. When you know that the Good Father is the God of your life you are surrendering your right to worry and to be anxious. He is the God of your everything; as Pastor Johnson has said, to worry is to take false responsibility for something. God is in control, He is the Good Shepherd. Know Him as such, and your paths will be made straight.

You might be thinking, "This is a nice Bible study, but what does this have to do with food?"

Everything.

Diets are our attempt to control our health and our body composition through using rules made up by mankind that have been applied to the masses.

God is also the God of your health, of your body, and of your nourishment. Do you trust Him there? Do you have an ongoing relationship with Him in each of those areas of life? Have you acknowledged that the One who created you wants you to live a life unhindered, with nothing standing between you and Him, and nothing stopping you from fully experiencing all that He has in store for you? God wants (far more than you will ever want) for you to be healthy, vivacious, joyful, thriving, and at peace with who you are.

He wants believers who live to celebrate the goodness of life.

Today, half way through, we ask that you take time to reflect on this idea. If it's on your heart, ask Him to show you what He wants for you in every area of your life. Yield to Him in all you do. Know that He is God.

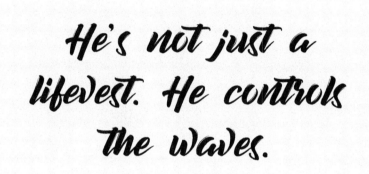

He's not just a lifevest. He controls the waves.

NOTES

AT THE KING'S TABLE

I WANT. HE FILLS.

Honing a Self-Controlled Thought Life

> "Finally, brothers and sisters, whatever is true, whatever is noble, whatever is right, whatever is pure, whatever is lovely, whatever is admirable— if anything is excellent or praiseworthy—think about such things."
>
> Phil 4:8

A self-controlled, Christ honoring thought life is key to the Christian life. In this broken world, we are surrounded by temptations. Fleshly desires can be overcome, but not if we allow the world to "corrupt" the condition of our minds. The enemy will use our thought life to destroy us by separating us from God. In his short time in the world, Christ wrestled with temptation as well. However, rather than thinking on that which tempted Him, he turned his thoughts to the Word and sought His Father's presence. Christ showed us the way to prevail over temptation. True, His sacrifice and resurrection washed us clean, but it also gave us the power of the Holy Spirit to prevail over temptation during our time in this broken world. Immersing ourselves in God's truth, allows His presence to guard and empower us to resist worldly temptations (1 Cor 10:13). Immersing ourselves in the Word takes our very thoughts captive and transforms them to Christ-mindedness.

Throughout the Bible, God gives us practical, "how to" instruction for honing a self-controlled, Christ honoring thought life. However, make no mistake, the enemy "prowls around like a roaring lion looking for someone to devour (1 Peter 5:8)." The enemy will constantly try to pry us from God's steadfast love and protection through an undisciplined, worldly thought life. He will use circumstances to disappoint, confuse, anger, and mislead. Each circumstance twisted inward to "why me?", gives rise to selfish desires. These desires open the door to worldly temptations. Although it is true, often, we cannot change the circumstance, however it is always true that God will use every circumstance for good. When we turn our thoughts to God, He leads us away from destructive inward thoughts and outward desires. He changes "why me?" to "how can this be used for His glory?" God's Word is armor against the plots of the enemy and our flesh. First, in Philippians 4:8, God instructs us how to flip the switch from self and the world to Him. In every moment (even our worst), Philippians 4:8 reminds us to think on all that is praiseworthy. To take our thoughts captive from what is false to all that is true, from the lowly to the noble, from wrong to right, from complicated to pure, from disagreeable to lovely, and from the inferior to the admirable. He instructs us to find all that is excellent and praiseworthy in our life; first of which is God. God is true, noble, right, pure, lovely, admirable, excellent, and praiseworthy. Philippians 4:8 commands us to think on God in the midst of every temptation, to invite Him into every circumstance, and to think as Christ: not on the trial but on the coming promise. By allowing our thoughts to focus on God, we are equipped to battle the enemy. Philippians 4:8 empowers us to move away from "why me" to "not my will, but Yours."

As well, God knew our pride would elevate the world's ways and stand in opposition to His truth; he knows the battlefield. In 2 Corinthians 10, God continues to equip us for victory while in the world. In verse five He instructs us how to turn away from the world's hypocrisy and conceit:

"take captive every thought to make it obedient to Christ."

In doing so:

"we demolish arguments and every pretension that sets itself up against the knowledge of God."

2 Corinthians 10:5 reveals the power of a self-controlled, Christ honoring thought life. Obedient thoughts not only protect us from temptation as detailed in Philippians 4:8, but Christ-mindedness can destroy worldly falsehoods before they take root. God continues to instruct in verses three and four:

"For though we live in the flesh, we do not wage war according to the flesh. The weapons of our warfare are not the weapons of the world. Instead, they have divine power to demolish strongholds."
2 Cor 10:3-4

Verse three and four reveal the fruitlessness of arming ourselves against temptation by through willpower or seeking worldly knowledge. Our power is not in our flesh. Reliance on the world empowers the enemy. Dependence on our flesh and the world strengthens their strongholds. Strongholds that will lead to death.

BUT GOD.

God, through His relentless, steadfast love and faithfulness, has given us "divine power" through spiritual weaponry that the enemy cannot withstand:

1. Know and speak the Word (2 Tim 3:16-17, James 4:8)
2. Declare the name of Jesus; remember the power of his name (Prov 18:10, Phil 2:9-10). He has overcome the world.
3. Put on the full armor of God (Ephesians 6)
4. Remember the power of prayer. (Romans 8:26) (Jeremiah 33:3)
5. Praise God, give thanks and corporately worship (Psalm 150)

Put on the full armor of God, Christ-mindedness demolishes every stronghold.

Remember: WE STAND IN VICTORY!

| LEADER-LED DISCUSSION:

- Take a recent circumstance in which you found yourself tempted, disappointed, frustrated, angry or misled and apply Phil 4:8 to flip the switch.
- How did Biblically reconditioning your mind change how you felt about the circumstance?
- In what areas do you seek the world's wisdom or your own powers without going to God first?
- How do these areas stand in comparison to the places where you are obedient to God?

| READING ASSIGNMENTS

John 16:12-15
1 Cor 2:11-16
1 Peter 4:1-2
Matthew 6:19-21
Luke 10:17-19

| SELF-CONTROLLED WARRIOR

The dictionary defines perseverance as:

> "Continued effort to do or achieve something despite difficulties, failure, or opposition."

The ability to keep moving toward any goal, despite setbacks and challenges, is a positive character trait. Indeed, it is one that we try to tap into for ourselves and instill in our children. Throughout the Bible we are called to persevere and given multiple examples of those that have. However, the difference between worldly perseverance and the Christian desire to develop a character of perseverance is found in who, how and why:

- In whom our confidence resides
- How we behave in the midst of trial (our attitude)
- Why we persevere

In Whom Our Confidence Resides

> "And I am sure of this, that he who began a good work in you will bring it to completion at the day of Jesus Christ." Philippians 1:6

As believers, we have confidence in our ability to persevere because God is working in, through, and for us. In other words, our confidence is not born of our own abilities, efforts, strengths or faith in self. Rather, we are confident in God: His saving grace, unconditional love, and desire for our good. When we doubt, falter, grow weary, or fail, He encourages and reminds us that He is steadfast. He is always with us. He is an endless supply of strength and a constant source of help:

> "Be strong and courageous. Do not be frightened, and do not be dismayed, for the Lord your God is with you wherever you go." Joshua 1:9

> "Fear not, for I am with you; be not dismayed, for I am your God; I will strengthen you, I will help you, I will uphold you with my righteous right hand." Isaiah 41:10

> "I can do all things through Him who strengthens me." Philippians 4:13

Believers persevere because we trust God's plan and will for our life (Jeremiah 29:11). When we submit to the truth that where we cannot, He can, we become self-controlled warriors. We confidently persevere no matter the circumstance or temptation because we have God.

| LEADER LED DISCUSSION:

- When difficult times or challenges come into our lives, where do you turn for comfort, strength and help?

Our Attitude in the Midst of Trial

> "Beloved, do not be surprised at the fiery trial when it comes upon you to test you, as though something strange were happening to you. But rejoice insofar as you share Christ's sufferings, that you may also rejoice and be glad when his glory is revealed." 1 Peter 4:12-13

The truth in our fallen world is that every person will encounter difficulties, challenges, and even tragedies that must be endured. However, unlike those without faith who often get consumed by feelings of frustration, anger, bitterness, and despair in the midst of adversity, believers are told "rejoice" and:

> "Count it all joy, my brothers, when you meet trials of various kinds, for you know that the testing of your faith produces steadfastness. And let steadfastness have its full effect, that you may be perfect and complete, lacking in nothing." James 1:2-4

Huh? Rejoice and "count it all joy" in the midst of trials? Neither Peter nor James suggest that trials and suffering are joyful: "fiery" and "testing". They understand that trials and suffering are trying, painful, and the cause of profound sadness. However, they know we can rejoice in the midst of our trials because faith "produces steadfastness." Faith reminds us that with Jesus we lack nothing and can "count it all joy"

Through our trials, whether merely frustrating or those that cause deep pain and suffering, faith reminds us that we are not of this world. The world's joy (happiness) is tied to circumstance and situation; it is fleeting because it's just an emotion. However, the joy of the Spirit (to which James is no doubt referring) is anchored in the truth: our hope is secured through the work of Jesus Christ. Peter's encouragement, as well, points to the eternal. Faith-filled joy is knowing not only are our valleys temporary, but we are not left to navigate them alone. We can rejoice and count it all joy in the midst of every trial because not only are we strengthened through Christ to persevere, but our trials draw us nearer to God and make us more like Christ:

> "We rejoice in our sufferings, knowing that suffering produces endurance, and endurance produces character, and character produces hope, and hope does not put us to shame, because God's love has been poured into our hearts through the Holy Spirit who has been given to us." Romans 5:3-5

| LEADER LED DISCUSSION:

- In the midst of difficulty or trials, do you pray "me prayers" or do you shift your focus to God and seek His purpose?
- What choices can you make to drink from the joy of the Spirit, focus on your blessings, and anchor yourself in eternal hope?

Why We Persevere

God's Word is clear that persevering through trials and enduring suffering are not requirements for salvation. Once trust is placed in Christ, salvation is secured. Our imperfect obedience is covered by Christ's sacrifice (His perseverance and suffering). God's saving grace cannot be earned; it is simply a gift, one on which we can depend, despite our bouts of doubt and unfaithfulness. However, we also know that trials are assured in a fallen world filled with broken people. So, if our salvation is secure, why should believers persevere and "count it all joy?"

- The ability to endure and remain anchored in the promises of God—to have an attitude of joy and rejoice in the midst of any trial—is one of the most powerful ways to witness and fulfill the Great Commission (Matthew 28:16-20).
- We trust that trials serve to deepen our walk with God. They prepare us for our eternal reward in Heaven by revealing the areas of our life that pull us from confidence in Him to fixation on self, areas we must give wholly to God to lean on His strength and find comfort in His love and peace. (2 Corinthians 4:15-18).
- Through our trials we are being shaped and conformed to the image of Christ and, therefore, they are for our good (Romans 8:28-30).

The decision to persevere in an attitude of joy is faith lived out; it is saying "Yes! I trust God's will for my life and believe ALL of His promises despite my circumstance." The character of perseverance is a cornerstone of mature faith: to keep your eyes fixed on your eternal hope and know you have everything you need in Jesus Christ.

We persevere because we trust God's faithfulness and His promises. Persevering with joy is the mark of an image bearer and makes us impactful seed planters. We persevere because, like Paul, we know the surpassing worth of knowing Jesus. We persevere because we live in this world confident in our eternal victory.

| LEADER LED DISCUSSION:

- We are warned throughout the Bible not to trust our own desires, in the false teachings of men, or worldly idols. In what trials do you turn to self, gurus, or seek comfort in the things of this world?
- How can you live out your faith through developing a character of perseverance? In what areas have you seen fruit from the decision to persevere?
- In trials you have endured, how did it strengthen your relationship with God? Were you able to not only surrender to "even if" but ask in its midst: "how can I be used to advance your Kingdom?" In other words, were you a seed planter and a light bearer?

| CONCLUSION

LEADER LED DISCUSSION:

- Open the floor to questions and ending discussion; set time cap if needed
- Set your next meeting day and time, if not already scheduled
- Close in prayer

READING ASSIGNMENT

- 1 John 5:14
- Hebrews 4:16
- Hebrews 10:36
- James 1:12
- James 5:11

Trust in the Lord with all your heart
and lean not on your own understanding;
in all your ways submit to him,
and he will make your paths straight.

Proverbs 3:5-6

WEEK 4
TRANSFORMATION
HABITS

FUEL YOUR BODY
EVERY MOVING THING
PROTEIN
FEED YOUR SOUL
JESUS. JESUS. JESUS.

"Everything that lives and moves about will be food for you. Just as I gave you the green plants, I now give you everything." Genesis 9:3

HABIT CHECK!

One of the best ways to feel full is to nourish your body in the way God intended. The Creator of all, including the miraculous machine that holds your soul and His Spirit, designed food specifically to fuel it well. As well, our Heavenly Father did not want our thoughts and emotions consumed by food. The food He created, when eaten in balance, quiets our body so our thoughts can focus on the Creator. We pray the foundation of a well-nourished body (hydrated and lots of vegetables and fruit) combined with a mindset focused on the provider rather than His provision are beginning to loose the binds of diet culture. Looking to God's plan to fuel your body and seeking Him first in this area, faithfully, will demolish the stronghold of diet culture. Continue to keep that foundation strong by consuming nutrient dense foods and renewing your mindset around consumption.

Remember: you have spent a lifetime adhering to diets and adopting a one size fits all lifestyle (yep, diets and every single "lifestyle" shares restriction and elimination as their foundation). Take the time you need to reinforce all that you have learned so you can finally be free to live your life: vibrantly, fully, and joyfully. You deserve all the time YOU NEED. You have permission to BE STILL and not move forward for a bit in this journey.

As always, we aren't going anywhere. And, God is faithful.

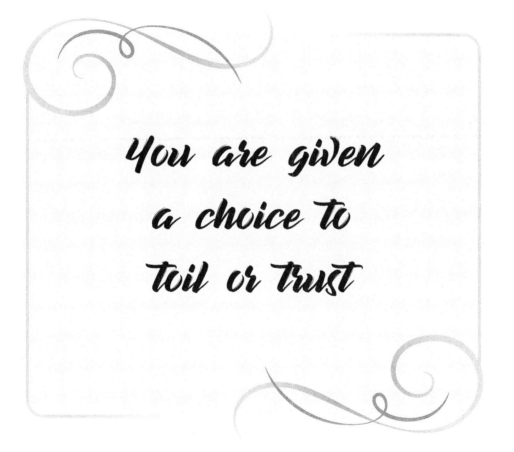

You are given
a choice to
toil or trust

EVERY MOVING THING: Protein

Week four begins the second half of this journey. We, of course, continue to build habits to nourish your body and renew your mind, but before diving in this week, might we suggest reading Romans. Paul reminds us in Romans 12:2 that in order to achieve a true transformation we must first renew the mind. Romans 12:2 is the foundation and goal of Break Through. Our prayer is that seeds are planted these six weeks to free you from a life consumed by fear and willfulness in your relationship with food. Seeds that take root, demolishing the stronghold of shame, so that your body is well-nourished and your spirit free from anxiety and worry in this area.

Today we're jumping into the first of the three macronutrients: Protein.

Protein is composed of amino acids, organic compounds that are the structural building blocks for life. Proteins can be classified as either essential (required in dietary intake), non-essential (produced in the body), or conditionally essential (may need to be supplemented by diet under special circumstances, like stress or illness).

When you consume protein it's broken down into amino acids which enter the bloodstream's amino acid pool. Here they're used to replenish cells of every type. In addition to providing structural components for muscle and tissue, amino acids are essential in producing hormones, neurotransmitters, antibodies, and enzymes.

A common misconception is that you must replenish protein stores immediately after exercise - in a 30-minute window of opportunity. This idea came from a series of studies on amino acid depletion following exercise that was being completed in a completely fasted state. Yes, if you are in a fasted state, your body is already depleted, and if you engage in strenuous exercise you further deplete your stores. In a fasted state, you do need to replenish your amino acid pool after exercise. If you are not in a fasted state (fasted state = no macronutrient- providing food or drink for at least 8-10 hours) when you engage in exercise, it is not necessary for you to drink a protein supplement or eat immediately following. The fact that this claim has survived through the years is largely due to supplement companies using it to sell their products. The body continues to synthesize protein for 48 hours following resistance training, and there is a period where the rate of breakdown in the body exceeds the rate of building (this is called a catabolic state), but if you've been eating well consistently your body will have enough amino acids in the bloodstream to counter the effects of catabolism.

You should, however, listen closely to your body and refuel accordingly. If you've eaten poorly or not enough in the day, you might want something fairly substantive after exercise.

| BENEFITS OF PROTEIN

Enjoying high-quality protein at meal times and with snacks has numerous health benefits. For one, protein is a thermogenic substance, meaning it actually increases your basal metabolic rate (BMR) a slight amount in order to digest and absorb the nutrients. It also helps to maintain a higher BMR by supporting muscle mass, which takes energy to simply maintain.

Consumption of protein also helps you to feel full and satiated by initiating a couple of key hormonal shifts. For one, it reduces the hunger hormone ghrelin. Not only does this provide an immediate sense of satisfaction, but studies also show that it pays off later in the day, too. In a study conducted in 2011, researchers found that adequate protein consumption (at least 25% of caloric consumption coming from protein) during the day reduced nighttime cravings and snacking by up to 60%. Protein also boosts blood levels of peptide YY, which helps you to feel full (recognizing fullness, a body that works for you rather than a body you must battle). You can consider protein a double whammy for normalizing appetite.

People often fear that an excess of protein can cause kidney damage. That is, for the most part, misplaced fear. If you have a pre existing kidney condition, then yes, too much protein can cause more harm than good. If this is you, please stick to the advice of your medical professional in determining protein consumption. If you do not have a kidney condition, then it would take an extraordinary amount of protein to cause actual harm to your body. It's highly unlikely that you are at risk of such issues.

How much do you need?

You can think about protein intake like an IV drip. You want a steady stream of relatively consistent amounts of protein throughout your day. And that's what today's habit is focusing on: creating consistency in protein intake and reaching adequate amounts of intake.

Today, we focus on the *general* guidelines to adequate protein consumption so that your body is well-nourished. Remember, our prayer is that you learn to nourish your body adequately so it stops battling you and consuming your thoughts. Adding all that is needed (abundance mindset) to be able to do all the things you like (exercise, playing with your children, living independently, pursuing adventure sports, serving others, etc.). Protein, because it is so filling, will also enable you to shift your focus away from food struggles; adequate consumption will help you focus on feeding your soul by deepening your relationship with God.

Women: Ladies, you know you need protein! But it's very likely that many of you undereat protein due to either media-driven fear of animal protein sources or simple taste preferences.

This week we challenge you to overcome those fears and to venture out into different recipes and preparation styles to find something that you genuinely look forward to eating.

The general guideline for adequate protein portions for women is as follows:

- Using the palm of your hand as a size reference, adequate protein is equal to one palm size serving per meal. As listed below in the "Tips For Getting Your Protein In" section, there are other options besides meat for your protein intake. We'll explain that in a bit.
- You should try to eat a total of at least 3-4 palm-size portions throughout the day but can likely tolerate up to 6 portions if you are consistently very active.
- If you're doing the math you probably realize that 4-6 palm- sized portions consumed one at a time at each meal means eating 4-6 times a day. Please note that you can, in fact, have protein as a snack. Also, we do not want to make you feel stressed to constantly be eating, so please be mindful of your natural hunger cues. We strongly believe that we all have different eating rhythms, and they may vary according to the day and time of the month. They may vary based on activity levels. Listen to your body and don't force it (honor hunger and recognize fullness over a forced consumption goal). The goal is to eat a a minimum of 3-4 portions so you are getting adequate protein.

Men:

- Using the palm of your hand as a size reference, measure out 2 palm-size portions of protein per meal. As listed below in the "Tips For Getting Your Protein In" section, there are other options besides meat for your protein intake. We'll explain that in a bit.
- You should try to eat a total of at least 6 palm-size portions throughout the day but can likely tolerate up to 8 portions if you are consistently active.
- As with the women, please listen to your body's natural hunger cues. If you are extremely active or have a high metabolism (or a lot of muscle mass) you may even want to go to 9-10 portions per day.

IT IS IMPORTANT TO DISCOVER YOUR BODY'S UNIQUE NEEDS SO THAT IT WORKS FOR YOU. GOD CREATED AND GAVE YOU AN INCREDIBLY ADAPTIVE AND BEAUTIFUL MACHINE: THROUGH CHRIST ALL THINGS ARE POSSIBLE!

CAROL + ALEX

| PROTEIN SOURCES

If it swims, flys, walks, or crawls, then it is yours to eat (Genesis 9:3). Animal meat will likely constitute the majority of your protein intake; therefore it is important to eat a variety of different sources to get the most nutrient benefits. For quality concerns, buy the best quality you can afford without allowing fear or anxiety to creep in. A good rule of thumb with all food purchases: higher quality choices for the foods you eat frequently.

If you dislike or have dietary restrictions that limit or eliminate animal meat, then know adequate protein goals can be met on a plant-based diet. However, it takes a bit more thought:

Plant-Based Protein: There are nine essential amino acids that the body requires but can't produce on its own. A primary concern for those eating either a strictly plant-based or nearly completely plant-based diet is that they don't get all nine essential amino acids in each day. The best way to ensure you're eating the right nutrients is by eating a wide variety of plant foods each day. There are "complete" plant-based proteins, meaning foods that contain all essential amino acids. Also, many plant-based eaters incorporate eggs and/or fish into their diet as well, both of which are complete essential amino acid sources.

Examples of plant-based protein sources:

- Quinoa: 8 grams of protein per cooked cup, a complete protein
- Lentils: 18 grams of protein per cooked cup, pair with rice for a complete protein
- Rice and Beans, together: A complete protein, with 7-10 grams of protein per cooked cup (this will vary according to rice:bean ratio, but this is an estimate

- Chickpeas: 15 grams of protein per cooked cup, pair with rice for a complete protein
- Hummus and Pita: Hummus is simply ground chickpeas, and pita contains all amino acids except lysine, which is found in hummus. So pair these two for a complete protein.

For ease, THINK: combine a grain and a legume to create a complete protein. If you choose veganism, then we encourage you to seek the assistance of a registered dietician to make certain you are getting all the nutrients you need.

Protein Supplements:

Protein supplements are an excellent (and tasty) way to get in a little extra protein. If eating your recommended amount of meat each day is proving difficult, you can replace one of those portions with a protein shake. Shakes are also a wonderful way to supplement a very active lifestyle!

Tips for getting your protein in

Meat and Eggs: As we mentioned, these will very likely constitute a good amount of your daily intake (unless you're plant-based). Good ways to ensure you have ready-to-eat meat on-hand include doubling your dinner recipes to have leftovers the day after, preparing protein in batches 2-3 days per week to keep in your fridge, and boiling eggs in batches to have on-hand. If you would like to carry your premade meat and eggs with you to work, we suggest getting a good cooler bag for storage. If you would like to substitute eggs for one of your palm-sized portions, ladies go for two whole eggs, and men go for 3-4 whole eggs.

Plant-Based: Again, variety is the key to getting in all essential amino acids each day. See the list in previous pages for complete protein combinations. Fortunately, it's relatively easy to make these foods in large batches, and they are easy to carry along with you.

Dairy: 1 cup of whole-milk plain Greek yogurt has 22 grams of protein. Women, we suggest 3/4 to 1 cup as a replacement of one palm-sized portion. Men, we suggest 1.5 cups to replace one palm-sized portion. 1 cup of whole-milk alone has just 8 grams of protein per cup. This is a good way to supplement your protein intake, but difficult to get an entire palm-sized serving worth of protein in at a time.

Supplements: Protein supplements account for one palm-sized portion. Men, feel free to add 1.5 or 2 scoops of protein to a shake if desired. We strongly advise having fun with your protein shakes and really amping up the flavor with some simple tips and tricks. A quick Google search will bring tasty recipes, like pumpkin pie protein shake, chocolate banana peanut butter protein shake, strawberries and cream protein shake, and more.

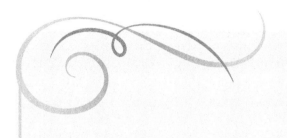

"And do not set your heart on what you will eat or drink; do not worry about it."

Luke 12:29

| REFLECTION:

Our prayer is to create awareness over adequate amounts of protein. Not enslave you to measuring or counting macros. Be mindful of your unique body's needs. Do not force or limit protein consumption to meet a goal. Entrenched diet mindset always leads to the binge/restrict cycle. Freedom from a toxic relationship with food is discovering the balance between what is needed and what is desired. When you meet your needs, desire lessens. Learn to listen to your body.

"Everything that lives and moves about will be food for you...."

SOME PROTEIN SOURCES

Beef	Poultry	Game
Brisket	Chicken	Bison
Chuck Roast	Turkey	Duck
Flank Steak		Elk
Ground Beef	Pork	Goose
New York Strip		Pheasant
Prime Rib	Bacon	Rabbit
Rib Eye	Boston Butt	Quail
Rump Roast	Ham	Thrush
Shank	Belly	Venison
Short Ribs	Chop	
Skirt Steak	Leg	Offal (Nose to Tail)
T Bone Steak	Loin	
Tenderloin	Shoulder	Blood
Top Round	Spare Rib	Crackling (pork skin)
Top Sirloin		Heart
Tri Tip		Kidney

Liver
Marrow
Oxtail
Sweetbreads
Tongue
Tripe

Other

Lamb
Goat
Mutton
Veal

Seafood & Shellfish

Amberjack
Anchovy
Bass
Bay/ Sea Scallops

Bronzino
Calamari
Catfish
Cod
Clams
Crab
Crawfish
Dorade
Flounder
Grouper
Haddock
Halibut
Herring
John Dory
Lobster
Mackerel
Mahi Mahi
Monkfish
Mussels
Octopus

Orange Roughy
Oysters
Pollack
Pompano
Salmon
Sardines
Sea Bass
Shad
Shark
Shrimp
Skate
Snapper
Sole
Tilefish
Trout
Tuna
Turbot
Whitefish

JESUS. JESUS. JESUS.

"But seek fIrst the kingdom of God and His righteousness, and all these things shall be added to you." Matthew 6:33

If Romans 12:2 is the goal of this program, then Matthew 6:33 is its cornerstone. Jesus called His followers to put their spiritual and eternal needs before the temporal things of this world. His teachings constantly emphasized placing the condition of your soul above your current circumstance. He knows that when you focus on your daily material needs or current situation, often the result is anxiety, pride, self-focus, shame, guilt, restlessness, bitterness, envy, and a need to be in control. The worries that come with putting the things of this broken world first are exhausting and life robbing. So each day, in every need and situation, you are faced with the choice to put your time and energy into the desires and things of this world or to invest in the kingdom of Christ and bring God glory. The command to seek first the kingdom is rooted in God's steadfast love for you. He knows with Him, in Christ alone, you have abundance: peace, contentment, rest, and joy.

In all things, Matthew 6:33 reminds you the choice is yours. You can choose to TOIL or TRUST.

Break free from the stronghold of toil

There are few areas of our life where we toil more than in our relationship with money or food. Diet culture has robbed us of our peace, contentment, rest, and joy with food. The enemy uses our self-reliance, envy, fear, appetite, and pride to imprison us in diet culture's falsehoods. We look to, and rely upon, it for answers. We not only DON'T seek God first in our relationship with food; we typically don't seek Him at all. Rather, we look inward to self or outward to the world of diet gurus, celebrities, social media, neighbors, mirrors, and scales. We look to anyone and anything that promises a quick solution to a body we dislike or promises rest from dis-ease. With each worldly falsehood we adopt, we are driven further from the protection and peace of God. We have become a culture that ceaselessly toils about food. We adopt diet after diet trying to find the lifestyle that won't leave us wanting and will deliver the goal we desire. We toil and empty our pantry of whatever is demonized by the latest trend. We become short-order cooks, cooking multiple meals to meet everyone's diet needs. Often, we discover the meals we feel forced to prepare and eat don't satisfy us, fueling frustration and appetite. The falsehood to control all things related to food also isolates us from fellowship. Our restrictions, eliminations, and food fears cause us to avoid social events and activities that will challenge our willpower. We allow our diet lifestyle to rob us of precious time with our Father through the constant demands of measuring, counting, and tracking. We beat ourselves up for "getting off track" or "falling off the wagon." With each new diet lifestyle, we toil more: we change everything about how, what, and when we eat. We toil in a quest for wellness. But, deep down we know it is anything but well with our souls.

Know this truth: the enemy seeks to destroy. He prowls like a lion, waiting for a way to use our current circumstance and worldly desires to separate us from God. Our desperate need for wellness has provided the enemy with the perfect opportunity, The world has twisted something that seems like a worthwhile pursuit into an obsession. We have been led far from God's protection in our relationship with food in an effort to achieve wellness. Food has become a source of anxiety, confusion, and shame. Worse, the more we diet and toil, the more our fleshly desires rule and lord over our lives. Our trust in willpower and diet culture has led to a life consumed by self-sufficiency and food. We have allowed how and what we choose to eat to steal our identity. The pursuit of wellness has become a false idol; it is an asherah pole of our time.

It's time to demolish
the asherah pole
of diet culture

Where the world gives us myriad ever-changing hoops to jump through and distracts us with hamster wheel toil, God's command is simple and unchanging: seek Him first in ALL areas of our lives. When we surrender to Him, trust Him, we receive all things. God's promise: when we SEEK HIM the brokenness of our flesh and the fallen world have no power. When we seek Him, we experience the fruit of the Spirit: love, joy, peace, patience, kindness, goodness, faithfulness, gentleness, and self-control. When we seek God first--in all things--we recognize that we are full with the abundant gift of Christ. We are empowered to let go of things we cannot control and equipped to battle the world's strongholds.

Seeking first the kingdom of God doesn't mean walking away from our responsibilities regarding family, work, school, or healthy pursuits. Rather, it means putting Christ first in our lives to protect us from our brokenness:

1. Ask: What am I prioritizing? In other words, where do you primarily spend your energy? Am I chasing the things of this world or am I serving others, spreading the Gospel, worshipping my Savior, and spending rich time in His word?

2. Seek: specific prayer for God to rule and reign in your life, in your choices; a God-centered life is not one of rules and regulations, but of righteousness, peace and joy in the Holy Spirit (Romans 14:17)

3. Surrender: a willingness to surrender your will to the will of God; an acceptance that what you believe you need is often different from what God knows you truly need. God will provide all that you need and protect you from all that you desire.

4. Share: When God "adds" to your life through the fruit of your more intimate relationship with Him, then use what

God has gifted to you or directed to you with others. Be a light for His kingdom. Shine brightly.

5.   Pray: "Take captive every thought to make it obedient in Christ" 2 Corinthians 10:5. You must strengthen yourself in the battle for your thought life. The enemy will tempt. Dive deep into the Word to arm yourself. The Holy Spirit has been given to you to HELP! Pray and listen. Allow the Holy Spirit to authentically transform you with His power.

Seeking first His kingdom does not mean that God will "fix" your life the way you most desire, but it will break you free from a life of purposeless toil, dis-ease, and the stronghold of shame. His promise is not to give you the body you desire, but a changed heart to know your body is a gift, beautifully made in His image. The eyes to see all that your body is capable of and the freedom to pursue His purpose for your life.

A life where you awake filled with hope, seeking His will for the day rather than someone consumed with the anxiety of "what am I allowed to eat; a life where your day ends praising Him for daily, abundant blessings; rather than one consumed with shame and remorse for the food choices you made.

> *"For the kingdom of God is not a matter of eating and drinking, but of righteousness, peace, and joy in the Holy Spirit." Romans 14:17*

The beauty of cutting down the Asherah pole of wellness and diet culture, you experience freedom. The more you turn away from life-draining, ever-changing rules of diet culture towards the peace of God, the less you will be ruled by cravings. Physically, restriction only enhances appetite and leads to binge behaviors. Spiritually, where you consider yourself weak in your inability to stay on track, God sees an opportunity to be in a deeper relationship with you. In your weakness, when you seek Jesus, God's power is made perfect. Look to Him. He is ever-present, faithful, and waiting to strengthen you. Make Him the greatest desire of your heart because His yoke is light. Run to the Cross and it will be well.

NOTES

AT THE KING'S TABLE

SPIRITUAL TOXINS

Toxic: adjective | \ täk-sik \ containing or being poisonous material especially when capable of causing death or serious debilitation

Just as we have the chance of being exposed to environmental toxins, we also run the risk of being exposed to spiritual toxins that threaten to undermine your faith and hinder your spiritual growth.

We are all broken. We all live within the inescapable confines of a fallen world. Every day the enemy prowls, looking for someone to devour. And 99% of the time, this devouring takes place over a matter of weeks, months, and years. It is not sudden, it is not obvious. The purpose of this lesson is not to point fingers but to hold you accountable to routinely do a self-check. Are you letting any of these things turn your eyes from God? Are you allowing these festering thorns to turn your heart from His?

> *"...keep yourselves in the love of God, waiting for the mercy of our Lord Jesus Christ that leads to eternal life." Jude 1:21*

In Jude, we are reminded that we have a ***responsibility*** to keep ourselves in the love of God. Notice the emphasis on the word "responsibility." God's love for us is unending, never-ceasing, and without flaw. He loves us, always. It is His intrinsic nature, not something that he chooses to do; love is who He is. But we have a responsibility to **keep ourselves** within His perfect and unfailing love.

Part of that responsibility is taking an honest look at our own personal culture and holding it up against the light of God's eternal truths.

| BITTERNESS AND RESENTMENT

Few things will erode away joy and harden a heart than the presence of bitterness and resentment. We've touched on this before, but it's worth saying again. Unforgiveness is toxic. Not only to your spiritual and emotional self, but also to your physical self. What takes root in the heart will affect the mind which influences the body. Your body can actually harbor physical manifestations of resentment and bitterness. It is an absolute urgency that you do a self-check to ensure you aren't holding on to unforgiveness or have a bitterness buried inside of you.

And sometimes we have to ask the Holy Spirit to help us with this self-check. Next time you have your time for prayer, ask Him to bring any unresolved resentment to light so that you can confess your unforgiveness and cancel all debts you feel this person owes you (even if that person is you). Forgiveness can be hard, especially when someone has done an unjustifiable wrong against you. Give all of your thoughts up to Christ, remembering that after He, the perfect, sinless lamb, had suffered unspeakable torture, pain, and humiliation, He forgave those who had crucified Him.

| ENVY

"Then I saw that all toil and all skill in work come from a man's envy of his neighbor. This also is vanity and a striving after wind." Ecclesiastes 4:4

We live in the age of #FOMO. The internet blasts us with all of the glamourous details of everyone else's lives on a daily basis. Being inundated with everyone else's affairs day-in and day-out is truly toxic. The quiet longing for the life and experiences of other people will set up camp in your heart, stealing your joy and destroying your full enjoyment of the life you have been given.

We strongly encourage you to keep a close eye on the thoughts going through your head when you're on social media or not - even if you think at first glance that envy isn't an issue for you, it could be hiding behind the curtain.

| YIELDING TO FEAR

Fear. Here it is again. Like unforgiveness, fear is such an overwhelmingly influential force that it's worth talking about again... and again... and again. It's no secret that God addresses fear repeatedly in the Bible, in fact it's mentioned over 360 times. God is well aware of the fact that yielding to fear will be a stumbling block for every person who walks the face of this earth. If not faced with a spirit of courage and boldness, fear will steal opportunity, rob dreams, and siphon potential.

Some kinds of fears are healthy. For instance, the fear that you feel when you watch your child do something risky is a healthy, protective, and a life-preserving fear. Likewise, fear can also keep you on-task and productive in your day-to-day schedule. Fear of being unnecessarily late for work, missing a deadline, or producing less than your best propels you to fulfill obligations and strengthen your abilities.

Fear can also act as an indicator that you are facing something new that will push you forward in some area of your life.

> "Fear is the guard dog that is protecting the fortress of spiritual prosperity. When the dog starts barking, we know that the treasure he is guarding is near." Pastor Johnson

The enemy works through fear most of the time. When he sees a child of God nearing something in life that will increase the child's spiritual prosperity and therefore threaten him and his agenda, he will use fear as a weapon to keep them from that "something."

And as we all know, some fears are unhealthy and undue. These fears (if left unchecked) will ultimately manifest themselves in crippling and paralyzing anxiety. These fears must be surrendered to the King of Peace. Go deep into His word and you'll find story after story of God's eternal peace stilling fears of all sizes.

Fear sewn by the enemy is toxic. If left unfaced, it will eventually seep into every area of life. Anxiety is a national epidemic in this day and age. As believers, we have the authority through the blood of Christ to rebuke every attack of the enemy. It's time we stand firmly in this authority and take back what the enemy has tried to destroy.

| SELF-SERVING THEOLOGY

This is a touchy topic, so please, hang with us. If your idea of God and how He works is inconsistent with His nature as is revealed in scripture, then you've created a self- serving theology in order to make sense of an issue in your life. And this is a mega toxin. God is who He says He is, so the question is, *do you know what He's said?* And we mean really know what He has said... The scriptures are in place to reveal God's nature to us. They contain stories that illustrate certain facets of His being and principles that lead to a righteous life. But the scriptures alone are not enough. The scriptures must be read *with the author at your side.*

The best way to understand the true meaning of scripture is to read a verse, then read it again. Reflect on what it is saying and consult with the Holy Spirit, asking for revelations of truth where needed.

We aren't saying that the Bible is cryptic. Far from it; it's accessible to any and all. But what we are saying is that as humans we can sometimes read the scriptures through a distorted lens, causing us to either misunderstand what it's saying or to only grasp a small portion of the truth being revealed.

And without the understanding of or even the familiarity of scripture, we are at risk of painting an inaccurate picture of who God is and how He operates. For instance, when someone is diagnosed with a serious or terminal illness, it is often human nature to make sense of that senseless tragedy by theorizing that it is God's will for their life. That is inconsistent with what we see in scripture.

In Matthew 10:8 we see Jesus commanding His followers to "Heal the sick, raise the dead, cleanse lepers, cast out demons..." just as He had been doing. And we know from John 5:19 that Jesus only did what He saw His Father doing. This reveals a very important facet of God's nature and desire for us: He wants all of us to be in perfect and divine health. So where does illness come from?

John 10:10 gives us a clue. "The thief comes only to steal and kill and destroy...". Anything that is adverse to the desire of God is an attack of the enemy. Plain and simple. Yes, God has ultimate authority. But we live in a fallen world, and adversity develops faith and perseverance that is necessary in order that we fulfill God's will for us here on earth: to usher in the Kingdom of God here on earth.

And John 10:10 continues with Jesus saying, "I came that they may have life and have it abundantly." That is the will of God. That will never, ever change.

| LEADER-LED DISCUSSION:

- Open discussion on spiritual toxins. Are there any questions? Does anyone have any input? Did we miss any toxins that may pose an issue for you or anyone in the group?

| READING ASSIGNMENT

- Romans 15:7
- 1 Corinthians 6:17
- Genesis 1:27

| SURRENDER

The Spiritual Discipline of Surrender

> "Therefore, I urge you, brothers and sisters, in view of God's mercy, to offer your bodies as a living sacrifice, holy and pleasing to God—this is your true and proper worship." Romans 12:1

Seeking the kingdom first, seeking the will of God above your own, and seeking His care, brings God glory and provides you with His peace. However, even a strong desire to be pleasing to God and knowing a better life comes from total surrender—*even* experiencing His peace in the areas that you are able to give to Him completely—does not make surrender the instinctive or easy choice.

Our time in the world is marked by the tension between flesh and Spirit; between our will and God's. Why? First, the word *surrender* immediately brings to mind the idea of sacrifice. It asks: what am I going to have to give up? Second, worldly culture confuses surrender with submission. In its view surrender is a sign of weakness: strong, successful people take control and are self-sufficient. Third, the enemy uses our fallen nature and a broken world to promote the lie that God keeps us from what is rightly deserved. Quite frankly, in the world, surrender feels wrong and is certainly not considered worthy. However, make no mistake, surrendering to God is not worldly! Despite the tension, how counterintuitive or difficult surrender is, God teaches that He is sufficient and desires nothing but our good. This truth is woven throughout the Bible.

The Old Testament is an account of willfulness and disobedience. However, in the midst of His justice, the Old Testament displays the depth of God's love. Despite their inability to surrender, God refuses to let His people go. The New Testament details perfect surrender through the life, death and resurrection of Christ. God willingly stepped down from Heaven, humbled himself and became flesh. He surrendered His own Son to redeem His people. Jesus surrendered to His Father's will. His choice to give all, gave *ALL*: forgiveness, His righteousness, freedom, peace, the Holy Spirit and a grave that cannot hold.

Surrendering completely to God, allows Him to work in you and through you; it allows you to experience the richness and depth of Christ's love. The more you surrender, the more you experience God's goodness. The more you surrender your mind, body and will to God, the more you discover His boundless mercy, His unending love and the sufficiency of His grace.

| LEADER-LED DISCUSSION:

- What are examples throughout the Old Testament of God's pursuit of His people.
- Give examples of lives fully surrendered to God in the Old and New?
- How is God's goodness experienced through their surrender?

The Path to Freedom: Total Surrender

> "I came down from heaven, not to do my own will, but the will of Him that sent me." John 6:38

Biblical surrender is willful acceptance of God's dominion over your life. Surrender is the decision to allow Him to direct your thoughts, to lead your actions, and to transform the desires of your heart; to desire Christ above all else. Surrendering to God, at its heart, is the choice to trust Him completely. When you surrender to God, you trust that His plan is for your good, His love is perfect, and your life is best used for His glory. Surrender is delighting in all that God desires for you: freedom from your brokenness and the burdens of this world. A surrendered life frees you from the pit of SELF and its reward of continual discontent. However, it is important to note, that surrendering to God does not promise a life without trial; rather, a surrendered life enables you to experience His peace in the midst of it. A surrendered life frees you to fulfill your Kingdom purposes. Surrendering all to God reveals the truth: with Christ we have EVERYTHING.

| A CHOICE: LOVE

> "This is how we know what love is: Jesus Christ
> laid down his life for us. And we ought to lay
> down our lives for our brothers and sisters" 1
> John 3:16

Jesus chose to completely surrender to the will of His Father. Christ's willingness to trust His Father's plan and His perfect love, conquered death and washed you clean. Surrendering to God is the choice to die to self to receive life. Making the choice to ask Jesus to lead your life and take residence in your heart, is a one and done proposition for salvation. However, daily surrender is choosing to look to God first in all things:

> "Father, if YOU are willing, take this cup from
> me; yet NOT MY WILL, but YOURS be done."
> Luke 22:42

When you yield completely to God, you experience the fullness of His mercy, love and grace. He wants abundance for you, but cannot fill what is closed. He longs for you to experience the depth of His love, to be joy-filled, to be free from fear, and to be fully satisfied. The more you give to Him, the more He is able to give to you. Choose to seek His will for your life and search out the areas you keep from Him. He faithfully waits, in every circumstance, for you to choose Him, to seek Him first, so that He can give you a life greater than you imagined.

| LEADER-LED DISCUSSION:

- Have you acknowledged that Jesus came to earth to live a sinless life that you cannot live, that He died in your place, so that you would not have to pay the penalty you deserve?

Have you confessed and invited Jesus to be the Lord of your life?

• If so, what is your current relationship with Christ like? In what areas do you need to choose to surrender more completely?

A heart that desires God in a world that desires self

"The king of Israel answered, "Just as you say, my lord the king. I and all I have are yours." 1 Kings 20:4

The path to freedom is a surrendered life, but few believers find all that God offers: a life free from fear, discontent, anxiety, and self. Most of us struggle with the fleshly desire to live for ourselves while having a heart that truly desires God. We desire to give *All......BUT*. By remaining tied to self and the things of this world, by storing up treasure, we limit God's ability to lavish us with His love because we deny Him our complete faith and love. As well, when we surrender with an eye on receiving a prize, we tell God we desire more, that His grace is not sufficient. Simply, no one can serve two masters. We cannot serve self and God. We cannot serve the world and God. When we are self-serving, we are not completely surrendered to God. He cannot completely free us from the burdens of our flesh or the world. BUT GOD. He, by His very nature, is faithful and patient. He relentlessly pursues us and calls to us to live out:

"I and all I have are yours."

He beckons us to trust that He is willing, able, and sufficient. He sacrificed His Son to pave the narrow way, sent His Spirit to guide our thoughts and hearts, and gave us His Word to know the truth of a surrendered life. He wants us to yield to His way so that we can feel the weight of our own will lifted. He wants us to be free of the burdensome yoke of this world and the enemy's strongholds. He wants us to fully surrender and to live solely for His glory! This is the path that God desires for all His children. He wants to fill our cups, provide us rest, enjoy His peace and love Him as He loves us.

> "For the Spirit God gave us does not make us timid, but gives us power, love and self-discipline."
> 2 Timothy 1:7

LEADER-LED DISCUSSION:

- In what areas is your surrender conditional? Are you giving Jesus the wheel, BUT keeping one eye or finger on it?
- If so, then ask yourself WHY? What fear, desire, or uncertainty keeps you from completely surrendering to His will for your life?
- In areas that you have fully surrendered to Him, what was your experience?

CONCLUSION

LEADER-LED DISCUSSION:

- Open the floor to questions and ending discussion; set time cap if needed
- For the next few weeks, we will unpack the spiritual discipline of surrender
- Set your next meeting day and time, if not already scheduled
- Close in prayer

Reading Assignments

James 4:7
Jeremiah 10:23
Matthew 26:39
Proverbs 23:26
Luke 9:23-24
Philippians 2:5-8

"But seek first the kingdom of God and His righteousness, and all these things shall be added to you."

Matthew 6:33

WEEK 5
TRANSFORMATION
HABITS

FUEL YOUR BODY
MANNA
CARBOHYDRATES
FEED YOUR SOUL
DEMOLISHING STRONGHOLDS

"Taste and see that the Lord is good; blessed is
the one who takes refuge in him." Psalm 34:8

HABIT CHECK!

If you haven't figured it out by now, we add what the body needs. A
well-nourished body is a body with healthy, trustworthy hunger cues
and diminished physical cravings. This common sense approach
reveals the dishonesty of diet culture. Rather than beginning with
all that needs to be added, diet culture demands restriction and

elimination. What they choose to restrict or eliminate does not matter (from calories to allowed times to eat). Restriction and elimination cause further nutrient deficiency, confusing hunger cues and increasing cravings. Restriction and elimination leads to only one place: over-indulgence and binge eating. Physical imbalances can never lead to a balanced relationship with food. Worse, despite the reality that restriction approaches are designed to fail (ok, 1.8% achieve sustainable success), most do not place the blame with diet culture. Rather, the constant cycle of failure leads most to the belief that they are out of control. Most become burdened with guilt and shame at their inability to be good. They judge themselves by the world's standards and their hearts harden towards the beauty of their bodies.

We pray you are adding in all the things a well-nourished, balanced body requires without falling prey to focusing on what you need to restrict. If you are well-hydrated, eating plenty of veggies and fruit, getting sufficient protein, then we bet you are feeling better and battling false hunger and cravings less. If you are continuing to shift your focus from yourself and the world to God, then we know the Spirit is revealing and convicting. We know a soul that is well-fed overflows with a peace that surpasses all understanding.

All this to say: keep adding God's good provision and God's goodness to your life.

*Imbalance
can never create
balance*

MANNA: CARBOHYDRATES

Considering how much angst carbs cause, most don't know what foods are classified as carbohydrates (outside of dreaded and demonized BREAD) nor what the function of carbohydrates are for our health and well-being.

| WHAT IS A CARB?

To put it simply, carbohydrates are a macronutrient, a primary source of energy for our body, and a crucial part of any well-balanced diet. Carbohydrates consist of three major components: sugar, starch, and fiber. They are classified as either simple or complex based on the number of sugar molecules and how your body processes them, but since many foods contain both it is often confusing to know what is what.

Simple Carbohydrates: one or two sugar molecules; rapidly digested.

Simple carbohydrates are made of basic sugars that are easily and rapidly broken down by your body. They can be an important source of energy when naturally occurring such as those found in fruit, vegetables, and dairy. However, the simple carbohydrates found in refined and manufactured food products, more often than not, lack nutrients. Without nutrients and fiber, they flood your body with sugar. When eaten in excess, simple carbohydrates that lack nutrients and fiber lead to hormonal imbalances, inflammation, mood, and energy swings.

So, the simple carbohydrates to be mindful of are those that are found in foods that lack vitamins, minerals, and fiber. Food products that have refined, added sugars such as baked goods, candies, soda, fruit juices, many cereals, many white flour breads, and chips as well as reduced fat dairy products, dairy alternatives, "health/diet" foods, canned fruits, and sauces flood your bloodstream with sugar. These simple carbohydrates can be enjoyed without guilt, but the amount and frequency of consumption requires mindfulness.

Complex Carbohydrates: longer chain of sugar molecules; slowly digested.

Complex Carbohydrates have, as you would expect, a more complex structure and are a rich source of vitamins, minerals, and fiber. These nutrient-dense carbohydrates take longer for your body to break down and; therefore, sugar is more slowly released. Rather than a flood of sugar followed by a crash (simple carbohydrates), complex carbohydrates provide a slow drip of energy at a more consistent rate.

Nutrient dense, complex carbohydrates such as true whole grains, legumes, and starchy vegetables are essential to satiety, health, and wellness.

SIMPLE ISN'T THAT SIMPLE

Naturally occurring simple sugars in complex foods

There are simple carbohydrates that naturally occur in fruit, vegetables, and dairy. Like all "basic" sugars, they are easily digested. However, because they are found within foods that are rich in vitamins, minerals and fiber your body absorbs and breaks them down more slowly (the higher the fiber content, the slower the release).

In short, the simple carbohydrates that naturally occur in nutrient dense foods function more like complex carbohydrates. These simple carbohydrates are essential to satiety, health, and wellness as well. Please do not let any diet or diet guru make you fearful of any vegetables or fruit; they need to be the foundation of your intake!

WHAT DO CARBS DO?

As we stated, carbohydrates are a primary source of energy for your body. Nutrient dense and fiber-rich carbohydrates:

- control blood sugar and insulin release - increase satiety and diminish cravings - maintain bowel regularity
- help reduce blood cholesterol levels
- improve brain function and clarity
- improve immunity and health of your GI system
- reduce the risk for numerous diseases, including heart disease.

Clearly, carbohydrates are a necessity for your health. Unfortunately, the food industry created a reliance on simple,refined carbohydrates. When our health declined and our waistlines increased, the answer was not a return to a balanced diet of nutrient-dense vegetables, fruit, and complex carbohydrates.

No. Diet culture demonized carbohydrates with a broad brush.

The tragedy: most people who fear carbs have walked away from fruit, starchy vegetables and whole grains (real food) and relied on diet culture products. Products that are often loaded with artificial sweeteners and lack nutrients.

THE POTENTIAL COST OF A LOW/ NO CARB LIFESTYLE

We will not argue the effectiveness of stripping weight off when you eliminate or drastically reduce carbohydrate intake. However, we will argue that your body was not designed for this artificial lifestyle. You are a complex machine that is intricately designed and one that relies on the energy (glucose) that carbohydrates provide.

After the short-term gains (well, loses) of a low/no carb lifestyle, the vast majority of us suffer disastrous health consequences (without addressing the elephant in the room: your ability to sustain the lifestyle for life and keep the weight off—you know, when your Keto friend states that they don't miss carbs for the 9th time, 10 minutes after you run into them—nor will we address the implications of diet culture demonizing "bread").

Some of the health consequences associated with a no carb/low carb diet:

- Decreased or impaired thyroid function
- Increased cortisol levels
- Moodiness and brain fog
- Decreased testosterone levels
- Suppressed immunity
- Lowered fertility
- Anxiety and depression
- Disrupted sleep and a decrease in quality sleep
- Chronic inflammation
- Imbalanced hormones, down-regulated metabolism (weight gain)
- Increased sensitivity to carbohydrates

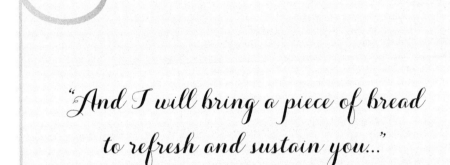

"And I will bring a piece of bread
to refresh and sustain you..."

Genesis 18:5

THE MILLION DOLLAR QUESTION: HOW MANY CARBS?

> "Then Jesus declared, "I am the bread of life. Whoever comes to me will never go hungry, and whoever believes in me will never be thirsty." John 6:35

Carbohydrate intake, like any other macro/caloric consumption, is not a one size fits all answer. (Keep in mind, when we are discussing carbohydrate intake we are focused on nutrient- dense, real food (fuel) carbohydrates). The balance of carbohydrates that an individual consumes is based on activity level and tolerance; it is highly individualized.

We do know that 70% of all people do well with an average carbohydrate intake; 25% fare better on a slight reduction in carbohydrates; 2.5% of the population (ultra-endurance athletes, etc.) need a higher intake of carbohydrates and approximately 1% of the population are keto adaptive. The small portion that remains are people that suffer from metabolic syndromes and optimal carbohydrate intake is based on their specific medical and health needs.

For now, let's focus on the necessity for sufficient carbohydrate intake to properly fuel your body and keep its functions balanced. For now, let's focus on putting down our fear of carbohydrates so they no longer take our thoughts captive.

> "We demolish arguments and every pretension that sets itself up against the knowledge of God, and we take captive every thought to make it obedient to Christ." 2 Cor 10:5

| BIG PICTURE

For the next week your goal is simple: disconnect from "carb derangement syndrome" by eating a balanced intake of nutrient-dense carbohydrates. In doing so, we will be able to reinforce eating sufficient vegetables & fruit while we stop fearing starchy vegetables, certain fruits, grains, and legumes. As we learned, these complex carbohydrates are necessary for our health and well-being. Let's learn the proper big picture balance (you know: getting an adequate amount).

For Women (single serving):

1 fist-sized portion of non-starchy vegetables
1 cupped palm size portion of starchy vegetables, fruit, grains, or legumes

For Men (single serving):

2 fist-sized portions of non-starchy vegetables
2 cupped palm size portions of starchy vegetables, fruits, grains, or legumes
Basic guidelines for adequate intake, any meals for inactive individuals or on days with no exercise (remember more activity requires more energy):

For Men and Women:

1/2 plate of non-starchy vegetables & fruit
1 cupped palm size portion or ¼ of plate of starchy vegetables, legumes or grains

Plant-based eaters, any meals:

1/2 of your plate is non-starchy vegetables
1/2 of your plate is a combination of legumes/grains, healthy fat 1 cupped palm size portion of fruit

You are meant for so much
more than a life imprisoned
by diet culture strongholds of
WHAT you are allowed to
eat or WHAT you weigh.

REFLECTION

Carbohydrate fear reigns supreme in diet culture; it has a grip like no other diet trend we have experienced (rather than fading; it mutates: elimination, gluten-free, cycling, fasting, net carbs and so on). Carbohydrate fear fuels the development and sales of artificial sweeteners and packaged "health" foods.

Despite knowing that our bodies require carbohydrates (yes, grain too) to function optimally, diet culture continues its assault on this macronutrient. What if the truth was simple? What if carbohydrates are not "bad" but our relationship with them is. What if we don't need to fear carbohydrates (or reinvent them), but respect their value. What if elimination and restriction are not the answer, but rather we must learn how to eat carbohydrates in respect to our bodies' needs kept in balance with our wants. Fear is a liar. Self-control is not an easy path, but it is a path of peace and one that leads to freedom.

We hope you occasionally indulge in—and truly SAVOR—your simple carbohydrate food passion. We hope when you do it is FREE of GUILT. We hope you have grown mindful of any physical cravings and are able to distinguish between hangry and hungry. Be mindful of any triggers from carbohydrate indulgences. Don't fear them, rather, learn how to effectively manage them. We hope with every food choice you empower self-control, moderation, and balance. We pray you are released from all food fears that rob you of joy, peace, and ultimately your health.

Our prayer is that you see the abundant value of a life focused on Jesus over food. Our prayer is that you are becoming impervious to a diet culture that markets to your fear and desire for easy. We want you free of food fear and false guilt. We want you to live a life that is no longer controlled by, or obsessed with food. We want you to stand firm in Christ and destroy every enemy stronghold that keeps you from your kingdom purpose. We want to disconnect you from the lure and lies of the latest diet trends and reconnect you to the TRUTH: You are meant for so much more than a life imprisoned by WHAT you eat or WHAT you weigh. We want you to lean into and upon the Holy Spirit: filled to overflowing with his goodness so that your life produces fruit.

| DEMOLISHING STRONGHOLDS

Food is a source of real pleasure: it tastes good, it is central to celebrations and traditions, it creates memories, and it provides comfort. At first food was solely associated with need. Babies sense hunger. Cry and are fed. However, it doesn't take long before eating for comfort comes into play. Slowly but surely, as we grew up, our relationship with food became far more complicated than just the filling of hunger needs. We received food as a reward for good behaviors. We were given food as a consolation. Unsurprisingly, food became less associated with physical need and more connected to emotional want.

Unfortunately, the already blurred line between need and want became further complicated with the creation of hyper-palatable food products and diet culture's ever- changing labeling of food as "good" or "bad." Foods' increased ability to trigger pleasure and diet culture's savvy marketing to tap into our deeply ingrained desire for anything restricted or forbidden has enslaved the majority of us in a toxic relationship with food. We WANT. We overeat. We restrict. We run out of willpower. We eat "bad." We feel "bad." We are drowning in the quicksand of dieting, shame, and guilt. The more we desperately struggle. The deeper we sink.

What is the healthiest transformation you can make? Drink more water and eat more vegetables? Sure. We love a shifted focus from deprivation to adding the fuel your body was designed to need. However, if your life is trapped in diet culture guilt:

BE STILL. SEEK THE KINGDOM.

The best thing you can do to heal your relationship with food and your body (and we would argue for your wellness) is to surrender one thing forever: the false guilt that comes from what you eat. False food guilt is a false guilt, a guilt that comes from the enemy. True guilt, guilt that comes from the Spirit, prompts you to repent and turn from sin. True guilt is met with forgiveness and grace; it is a choice made but not one to which you are lost. True guilt shifts the focus from your actions to the solution: JESUS. True guilt leads you to meditate on the truth in God's Word:

> "As far as the east is from the west, so far has he removed our transgressions from us." Psalm 103:12

False food guilt and the stronghold of shame has stolen so much precious time from Jesus.

False guilt is a weapon of the enemy with one purpose: to tear you away from your relationship with God.

Truly, ditch the guilt. Beating yourself up about something you ate is not only futile (you cannot un-eat it) it is insidious. False food guilt is the tiny whisper: no matter what you do, you will fail and your failure is unforgivable. False guilt destroys because it leads to shame. The place where what you do becomes who you are. Shame is an enemy stronghold. False guilt ensnares your mind, keeping you focused on yourself and what you desire. It is not a mindset that looks to Spirit empowerment and self-control. No. It is a life lived in the enemy strongholds of willpower and shame. And, it is destructive.

False food guilt accepts the premise that there are "bad" foods and if you consume them, then you are "bad." Think of the language used by diet culture: cheater and unclean. Even worse, the enemy not only deceives to ensnare he twists. The list of foods that make you "bad" constantly changes and grows: eggs, butter, dairy, sugar, fat, gluten, meat, lectins, carbohydrates, bread, bananas, legumes, nuts, anything cooked, processed, packaged, anything with a face, tuna, any fruit besides berries, white potatoes, white rice, canola oil--no coconut oil, wait corn oil...oh, corn, and anything eaten before noon. False food guilt is no longer associated with Twinkies (and, let's face it Twinkies don't make you a "bad" person). Now, you are filled with guilt and shame for eating too much fruit, the wrong vegetable, and Heaven forbid if you forget yourself and eat BREAD. False food guilt and shame, combined with an ever changing list of what is "bad", has stolen so much precious dependence and time from Jesus.

> "Look at the birds! They don't worry about what
> to eat--they don't need to sow or reap or store up
> food--for your heavenly Father feeds them. And

you are far more valuable to him than they are."
Matthew 6:26

Here are just a few of the bitter fruits that are reaped from a life lived in the stronghold of False food guilt and shame:

- Private/shame-filled eating
- Binge eating/throwing in the towel
- Self-denigration: we are fat, weak, lazy, out-of-control
- Judgement of others
- Food obsession (allowed, forbidden, when, how much)
- lost fellowship
- lost freedom and peace that comes from Spirit-led self-control
- lost joy of exercise as it is twisted into punishment for "bad" food choices or a joyless necessity to be allowed to eat something

Finally, if all that is not enough destruction, the enemy uses our False food guilt and the stronghold of shame to make us feel unworthy of seeking the Kingdom. Eventually, how we eat begins to claim our identity: Keto, Vegan, Gluten-free, Carb-cyler, Intermittent Faster, Clean eater....

HOW YOU EAT IS NOT WHO YOU ARE.

YOU ARE HEIR TO THE KINGDOM. A CHILD OF GOD, LOVED, FORGIVEN, TREASURED, AND PURPOSED.

"I praise you, for I am fearfully and wonderfully made. Wonderful are your works; my soul knows it very well." Psalm 139:14

False food guilt imprisons you in the enemy stronghold of shame with one purpose: draw you far from God's truth and protection. Only through an intimate relationship with God can our minds be renewed, our lives transformed. Only through Christ can we have the strength to be self-controlled warriors. Ones who are not ruled by our flesh.

Nail False food guilt to where it belongs: the cross.

| PRO TIPS:

Awareness: Become aware of your negative food language: "cheat day" "cheat meal" "allowed" "forbidden" "bad" "junk" "cheat food" "naughty" "clean" "guilty pleasure" "sinful" "my weakness" "reward meal" "how many carbs" "unhealthy" "toxic" "how many calories" "what is the cost" "I shouldn't" "I'll pay for this" "I'll eat this now, but will (exercise, skip a meal, be better tomorrow, etc.)" "I don't miss it" "I can't have it again until" "I can't believe I ate that" "I'm weak" "I have no willpower" "Why even bother" "I'm hopeless" "I have no self-control" "I need to burn this off" "No carbs for me for a week". When you grow aware, you can choose to stop negative food language in its tracks.

Stop labeling: Food is not "bad" or "sinful". You aren't "cheating" when you eat. Labeling food (and yourself) in a negative way gives food power that it simply does not deserve; agonizing over and micromanaging every bite you take is unhealthy. Food has a purpose: to fuel and nourish our body, to fill an emotional, social or situational need.

Retrain yourself instead of restraining yourself: Ask yourself WHY you are about to eat something that triggers False food guilt. If the reason is emotional, eat it or leave it.

[a] If you choose to eat it, then please ENJOY it guilt free. You are more likely to eat a balanced amount of it (a slice of cake, rather than the whole cake, licking the icing off the plate and then digging through the trash to get the part you threw out in disgust). Savor it, chewing slowly, rather than wolfing it down wracked with guilt.

[b] If you choose to leave it because you know you aren't hungry, but you have an emotional need then fill, then take that need to God: Pray. Read the Word. Praise and Worship him. Remember, we were trained as children to comfort ourselves with food. Food, however, does not provide lasting comfort. What does: a rich, intimate relationship with God.

Honor your body: If you are about to eat something that triggers False food guilt, but you are actually hungry, then take a moment to unearth the need. Hunger means their is a physical need. Have you eaten enough today or did you skip a meal? Have you eaten enough vegetables, fruit, protein, fats, etc. We've spent so long ignoring our bodies' needs, we no longer honor them. We've spent so long restricting foods because we believe them to be "bad", that we've created real nutrient gaps.

Grace: If you are consumed by negative food language, then chances are you are deep in diet culture quicksand. False food guilt has power over you and is in control. Relax your restrictions. Chances are your willpower is diminishing as your deprivation grows louder. Remember we are hardwired to desire that which we are denied. What is not allowed becomes all we crave. Chances are, in today's diet culture, you are restricting real nutrient needs as well. So you are not only hangry, you are hungry. Show yourself some grace and remind yourself that no one eats perfectly. Life happens. Perfect isn't possible and what is considered "perfect" changes daily in the world of nutrition. Chasing perfection is exhausting and unhealthy. Rather, seek a relationship with food rooted in Spirit-led self-control. One free from negative False food guilt labels. Food either fuels your body or feeds your soul. Figure out which you want: nourishment or pleasure. Give yourself permission to eat.

Break Free: Walk away from diets. All restrictive diets reinforce negative food language (they just change which foods they label as "bad"). If we remain a prisoner to any diet, then we will eventually "fall off the wagon" and eat the "bad" food. Remember, False food guilt fuels diet culture's bottom line and strengthens the enemy's strongholds. Surrender this area of your life to God!

> "Do not be anxious about anything, but in every situation, by prayer and petition, with thanksgiving, present your requests to God. And the peace of God, which transcends all understanding, will guard your hearts and your minds in Christ Jesus." Philippians 4:6-7

NOTES

AT THE KING'S TABLE

GIVE US THIS DAY

| WHAT YOU HAVE, WHAT YOU NEED

"After this Jesus went away to the other side of the Sea of Galilee, which is the Sea of Tiberias. And a large crowd was following him, because they saw the signs that he was doing on the sick. Jesus went up on the mountain, and there he sat down with his disciples.

Now the Passover, the of east of the Jews, was at hand. Lifting up his eyes, then, and seeing that a large crowd was coming toward him, Jesus said to Philip, "Where are we to buy bread, so that these people may eat?" He said this to test him, for he himself knew what he would do. Philip answered him, "Two hundred denarii worth of bread would not be enough for each of them to get a little." One of his disciples, Andrew, Simon Peter's brother, said to him, "There is a boy here who has five barley loaves and two fish, but what are they for so many?" Jesus said, "Have the people sit down."

Now there was much grass in the place. So the men sat down, about five thousand in number. Jesus then took the loaves, and when he had given thanks, he distributed them to those who were seated. So also the fish, as much as they wanted. And when they had eaten their fill, he told his disciples, "Gather up the leftover fragments, that nothing may be lost." So they gathered them up and filled twelve baskets with fragments from the five barley loaves left by those who had eaten. When the people saw the sign that he had done, they said, "This is indeed the Prophet who is to come into the world!"

Perceiving then that they were about to come and take him by force to make him king, Jesus withdrew again to the mountain by himself."

John 6:1-15

Bread is mentioned at least 492 times in the Bible. It symbolizes sustenance and provision, a token of God's attention to our most basic needs. It is certainly not made to be something to be feared. Interestingly enough, it is actually portrayed to be something to be respected. It is recognized for its life-supporting qualities and as a blessing from God. Let *that* sink in.

Here in the first fifteen verses of John 6 we see the well-known story of Jesus using a boy's grocery haul of five loaves of bread and two fishes to feed a crowd of 5,000. (Interestingly, this is the only story of Christ's *life* that is recorded by all four gospels.)

In the story, it is around Passover time and the hungry crowd had gathered to hear Jesus speak. When Jesus saw the size of the crowd he first turned to Philip, who expressed concern over being able to feed them all. *"Where are we to buy bread, so that these people may eat?"*

Philip asks anxiously. Now let's pause here. In the second chapter of John we see Jesus at the wedding feast at Cana with his disciples, Philip included. Philip watched with his own eyes as Jesus turned water into wine (and not just any ol' wine; it was the finest wine at the feast). So, what's happened? Did Philip suffer a head injury sometime between the wedding and the feeding of the 5,000? How could he ever question the ability of Jesus to provide after witnessing his first miracle?

Philip, like all of us have done at some point(s) in our lives, doubted Jesus's ability to provide because he was looking through the lens of earthly reality. How different would Philip's reaction to the situation be if he had instead looked through the lens of kingdom possibility?

And Jesus, being both fully man and fully God, acted out of kingdom reality and took *what they had* and made it *more than enough*. When you hand Jesus what you have, do you have the faith to believe that He will make it what you need? With a little extra for good measure?

We aren't orphans at an orphanage, our basic needs being supplied by a headmaster. No, we are children of a good Father who delights in not only providing for us but in also satisfying our dreams and desires. *(Sometimes a delay in answer can be confusing; but remember, God will never answer a prayer if it means undermining His purpose for you here on earth.)*

Never pay more respect to the size of your problem than the size of your God.

| LEADER-LED DISCUSSION:

- Open the floor for discussion about faith in provision. What areas of life do you freely entrust to God? Which do you hold on to with clenched fists? Why not trust God with your all?

| GIVE US THIS BREAD, ALWAYS

"Our fathers ate the manna in the wilderness; as it is written, He gave them bread from heaven to eat. Jesus then said to them, "Truly, truly, I say to you, it was not Moses who gave you the bread from heaven, but my Father gives you the true bread from heaven. For the bread of God is he who comes down from heaven and gives life to the world." They said to him, "Sir, give us this bread always."

John 6:31-34

For the bread of God is *He* who comes down from heaven and gives *life* to the world. Our sustenance is found in Jesus alone. He is, as He's quoted saying in John, the bread of life. All who come to him will never be hungry again.

How have we come so far as to arrive at a point in time when bread could be seen as something that is to be avoided? A number of reasons come to mind, but the demonization of bread by diet culture is most notable. But that belief is of this world. God loves to talk to us through winks. Small, subtle flashes of His beauty in the natural world happen every day: the rainbow after the storm, the butterfly outside your window, the birds in the morning, the frogs at night. Who are we to say that a simple loaf of freshly baked bread that fills the house with the aroma of *enough* and provides your body with the energy to *do* isn't an intentional reminder of God's gift of Christ, the bread of life?

We think it is, and we won't let the fear and confusion of the world take that God wink from us. God is in the details of the everyday just as much as He is the author of all that has been or will be. Yes, Lord, please give us this bread *always*.

| LEADER-LED DISCUSSION:

- Open the floor for discussion about the legitimacy of fears, be it related to food or other. How often does the author of confusion and fear (the enemy) blind you to the subtle God winks?

| READING ASSIGNMENT

- Job 37:14-16
- Psalm 19
- Psalm 95
- Romans 1:20

| DEMOLISH STRONGHOLDS

Guilt is a tricky emotion. When the source of guilt stems from our desire to be pleasing to God, it is spiritually anchored and enriches our faith walk. However, the vast majority of guilt felt is of this world; it is false guilt and its enemy led. This guilt is born of fear and leads to the stronghold of shame. False guilt pulls us further from the protection of God's love. Simplistically, there are two types of guilt:

- God-sparked guilt: restorative
- Enemy led false guilt: destructive

    "Godly sorrow brings repentance that leads to salvation and leaves no regret, but worldly sorrow brings death." 2 Cor 7:10

| GOD-SPARKED GUILT

God-sparked guilt is not focused on self. Rather, it is born of a God who desires us (2 Peter 3:9) and wants to protect us without usurping our will. God-sparked guilt is an inward sign of His relentless pursuit of us:

> "I myself will be the shepherd of my sheep, and I myself will make them lie down, declares the Lord God. I will seek the lost, and I will bring back the strayed, and I will bind up the injured, and I will strengthen the weak." Ezekiel 34:15-16

Fallen, we stand guilty before a Holy God with no ability to reconcile and be with Him. Neither our actions or thoughts can wipe us clean. However, His love for us is so complete, and His desire to reconcile with us so great, that we feel His pull. God- sparked guilt is the quiet knock on the door to our hearts. It beckons us to turn from the world and to trust Him, receive His grace and, in that, be fully reconciled:

> "Behold, I stand at the door and knock. If anyone hears my voice and opens the door, I will come in to him and eat with him, and he with me." Revelation 3:20

Once reconciled, God-sparked guilt continues to convict us: it is a gentle correction, an internal compass leading us home. When we feel God-sparked guilt, we recognize our disobedience, acknowledge our weakness, and feel our constant need for Jesus. This guilt is not a weapon used against us; rather, it is for our good. God-sparked guilt does not cause us to feel shame. In fact, it creates the exact opposite feeling: It is a reminder that, despite our brokenness, we are of such worth to our almighty and loving God, that He sacrificed His only Son for us. God-sparked guilt doesn't draw us further from His love, it holds us in His hand:

- It leads us to repent
- It reminds us to submit to His will
- It strengthens and enriches our faith walk

Our repentance is an outward sign of God's victory! God-sparked guilt leads to justification and it is the Holy Spirit's continued work to conform us to the image of God's Son (Titus 3:5).

| LEADER-LED DISCUSSION:

- God-sparked guilt is directional. It is the spirit leading us to God and securing our lives in His hand. How does this guilt drive you towards reconciliation and restoration?
- Do you recognize that God-sparked guilt is a symptom of God's love?

| ENEMY LED FALSE GUILT

If God-sparked guilt leads to salvation and is transformative, then where does enemy led guilt lead? First, however, we must look to a source of false guilt. Often, guilt is the result of choices made against what we know to be right. Guilt, then, can be a useful tool to draw us back to the narrow path. However, often in a fallen world, rather than leading to repentance, false guilt becomes anchored in self. This type of guilt is the enemy's weapon. He uses it to fuel fear and feed pride:

- we don't measure up
- we deserve more...so our actions are justified
- it wasn't our fault

- if I get caught how will I be negatively impacted

Enemy led false guilt does not seek the healing and redemptive power of God; rather, it causes us to fixate on our own needs and our own hurt. We make ourselves our own idols and boast in our own power. This is a destructive path.

Enemy led false guilt whispers: you are not worthy, strong enough, rich enough, good enough or attractive enough. False guilt uses our brokenness to keep us in an endless vortex of self-desire and imprisoned within the stronghold of shame. False guilt places our desires and will above God's, seeking our own glory and trusting in our strength. This pride leads us to place our faith in works. Our hearts harden against God. With our faith in works, the enemy uses our failings to trap us in the stronghold of shame. Shame whispers: "you cannot earn God's forgiveness so why bother." False guilt is born of the lie: that we can earn God's love. Enemy led false guilt leads to death.

> "You felt secure in your wickedness. 'No one sees me,' you said. But your 'wisdom' and 'knowledge' have led you astray, and you said, 'I am the only one, and there is no other.'" Isaiah 47:10

| LEADER-LED DISCUSSION:

- In what areas of your life do you become trapped in the vortex of self-desire and the stronghold of shame?
- How would things transform if you placed your trust completely in God and sought Him and His counsel?
- What are practical ways you can seek God's truth in these areas?

| THE GOOD NEWS

False guilt is the enemy's weapon to separate you from God. But God relentlessly pursues what is his. No matter your sin, the weight and noise of your false guilt, God-sparked guilt is quietly whispering: come home, you are worthy, you are loved and my grace awaits you:

- God has done what you cannot. (Romans 8:3)
- Your guilt has been nailed to the Cross. (Colossians 2:14)
- Christ's sacrifice replaced your guilt with God's righteousness. (1 Peter 2:24)
- This is the free gift of grace and the good news of the Gospel. (Romans 6:23)

All you need do: open your heart, acknowledge your guilt and trust in Christ's sacrifice. Acknowledge that no works can acquit you before a Holy God. Rather, his love is so perfect that he freely became flesh, suffered, died your death, and rose from the grave. Jesus's sacrifice made you right before a Holy God and clothed you in righteousness. He loves you and calls you worthy. His mercy is infinite. His forgiveness and grace are free. Turn away from the world and trust in Jesus.

Set your ear to the whisper of God-sparked guilt because it is God's relentless pursuit of you. He desires nothing more than for you to come home.

> "What do you think? If a man has a hundred sheep, and one of them has gone astray, does he not leave the ninety-nine on the mountains and go in search of the one that went astray? And if he finds it, truly, I say to you, he rejoices over it more than over the ninety-nine that never went astray. So it is not the will of my Father who is

in Heaven that one of these little ones should perish." Matthew 18:12

LEADER-LED DISCUSSION:

- If the enemy uses false guilt to separate you from God, in what ways has God relentlessly pursued you and washed you in His grace?
- If you feel moved to lead a salvation prayer for your group, then have them repeat after you:
- "Dear Lord Jesus, I know that I am a sinner, and I ask for Your forgiveness. I believe You died for my sins and rose from the dead. I turn from my sins and invite You to come into my heart and life. I want to trust and follow You as my Lord and Savior."

CONCLUSION

LEADER-LED DISCUSSION:

- Open the floor to questions and ending discussion; set time cap if needed
- Set your next meeting day and time, if not already scheduled
- Close in prayer

READING ASSIGNMENT

- Titus 3:3-7
- 2 Chronicles 7:14
- Jeremiah 29:11-14
- Ephesians 2:8-9
- Revelation 5:9
- Romans 5:3-5

"For though we live in the world, we do not wage war as the world does. The weapons we fight with are not the weapons of the world. On the contrary, they have divine power to demolish strongholds. We demolish arguments and every pretension that sets itself up against the knowledge of God."

2 Corinthians 10:3-6

WEEK 6
TRANSFORMATION
HABITS

FUEL YOUR BODY
FAT OF THE LAND
FATS
FEED YOUR SOUL
FROM FEAR TO PEACE

HABIT CHECK!

Carbohydrates are so demonized by diet culture; yet, such a necessary fuel for your body. We pray this last week has given you greater insight into carbohydrates and that no vegetable or fruit is to be feared! We pray this last week has revealed the stronghold of False food guilt and you have begun the work to free yourself from diet culture's shame cycle. As we begin the final week, we pray the foundation of your intake is vegetables and fruit (carbohydrates) because a well-fueled body works for you: sufficient intake of micronutrients and fiber normalizes hunger cues and reduces cravings. We pray you understand that foods (ANY FOODS) that provide comfort or are the stuff of celebration and fellowship can be enjoyed without guilt. For our fuel habit, this week is dedicated to the last of our three macronutrients: fats. We end our feed your soul habits with shifting from diet culture's fear mindset to Kingdom peace. Foods' purpose is to fuel our body, but God--because he is good--gave us tastebuds, dopamine hormones, and delicious things to eat. All food can be enjoyed without falling prey to overindulgence.

> "Do you like honey? Don't eat too much, or it will make you sick!" Proverbs 25:16

> "And do not get drunk with wine, for that is debauchery, but be filled with the Spirit," Ephesians 5:18

| FAT OF THE LAND: FATS

WHAT IS DIETARY FAT?

The stuff that we know as dietary fat consists of fatty acids, the simplest unit of structure in fat molecules. A fatty acid is a simple hydrocarbon chain (chain composed of hydrogen atoms and carbon atoms) with signature groups attached to each end of the chain. When the actual structure of the chain between those signature groups changes just slightly, we see a different type of fatty acid that will behave differently in biological environments.

The first type of fatty acid is the saturated fatty acid. These are called saturated because there are no double bonds between carbons in the chains, meaning that as many hydrogen atoms as possible are attached to those carbons. Hence we have the name "saturated." Because of their structure, saturated fat is often solid at room temperature.

Examples of saturated fat sources:

- Animal meat including beef, poultry, pork
- Certain plant oils such as palm kernel or coconut oil
- Dairy products including cheese, butter, and milk
- Processed meats including bologna, sausages, hot dogs, and bacon
- Pre-packaged snacks including crackers, chips, cookies, and pastries

Saturated fat has been thought to be less healthy for the human body, although those findings are coming under scrutiny now as more research is disproving those claims. The previous studies arrived at the conclusion that saturated fat may lead to higher levels of LDL which can increase an individual's risk for heart attack or stroke. However, new research is showing that other things might actually be to blame, like consuming too many processed foods and simple sugars. As you can see in the above list, many foods that contain saturated fats are also highly processed. Our take on saturated fat from wholesome ingredients and real food is simple: everything in moderation.

When a fatty acid chain has one or more double bonds between carbon atoms and there are fewer hydrogen atoms than possible, that is called an unsaturated fatty acid. Unsaturated fatty acids are usually liquid at room temperature, which makes sense considering they have fewer hydrogen atoms to give them a rigid structure.

Depending on how many double bonds exist in the hydrocarbon chain, unsaturated fat can be classified as either monounsaturated (one double bond) or polyunsaturated (more than one double bond).

Examples of unsaturated fat sources:

- Nuts
- Plant oils such as vegetable oil
- Certain fish like salmon, tuna, and anchovy, which contain
- omega-3 unsaturated fatty acids
- Olives
- Avocados

Research has always indicated that unsaturated fats have a positive impact on your health. But as with everything, always consume in moderation and according to the general portion guidelines we will be giving you later in this lesson.

One type of polyunsaturated fat is particularly important, and that is the Omega-3 fatty acid. In case you are wondering, the name "Omega-3" tells you a little about the structure of the hydrocarbon chain. What this is saying is that the final double bond between carbon atoms sits at the third carbon atom from the Omega end (the methylated end) of the fatty acid chain. So the little dash between the two is actually a "minus" indicating 3 carbons *from* the Omega. That's wayyyy more than you need to know, but if you wanted to know, then there you go.

"What we don't understand, we fear. What we fear, we judge as evil. What we judge as evil, we attempt to control. And what we cannot control... we attack."

– author unknown

So what's special about these Omega-3's? They have potent anti-inflammatory properties and work to counteract the pro-inflammatory actions of the closely related Omega-6 fatty acids (pop quiz: where is the final double bond located in an Omega-6 fatty acid?). The standard diet today contains an excess of Omega-6 fats and a deficit of Omega-3 fats. You can see how the scales can start to tip over time, leading to chronic illness and metabolic dysfunctions.

Foods high in Omega-3 fats:

- Salmon
- Cod liver oil
- Flaxseeds
- Chia seeds
- Walnuts
- Coconut oil

If three fatty acid chains come together with a glycerol molecule, we have a triglyceride. This type of fat is the primary form of fat in the diet and the primary form of fat that gets stored in the body. When you consume in excess, that unneeded energy is converted into a triglyceride which then circulates in the blood and can be stored as fat. When the body needs to burn triglyceride stores, it breaks the triglyceride down into its component parts - three fatty acids and a glycerol molecule - for use as energy.

Finally, we have trans fats, which are primarily found in processed foods and refined, hydrogenated oils. As you probably know, these trans fats have been determined by peer-reviewed, medical research (not "cherry-picked" diet research) to be detrimental to overall health and, therefore, need to be eaten mindfully and rarely.

Common sources of trans fats:

- Many brands of cake mixes and store-bought frosting
- Many brands of frozen biscuits
- Microwaveable meals, especially breakfast sandwiches and the like
- Margarine
- Cream-filled candies
- Some store-bought donuts
- Many brands of frozen pizzas
- Many brands of crackers and chips

DIETARY FAT VS. BODY FAT STORES

Dietary fat does not automatically mean body fat. We believe it's fair to say that most people have come to the point where they no longer fear fat (but how many remember the "fat-free" craze), but just in case let's look at some of the very important roles that dietary fat plays in supporting bodily processes.

- They make the body go! Fat is the most energy-dense macronutrient, carrying 9 kilojoules (or calories) of energy per gram consumed. This isn't a reason to fear fat, but rather, it's a reason to respect fat.
- They provide structural integrity to our cells. The membrane of cells is made up of phospholipids, triglycerides, and cholesterol. These membranes are truly amazing, as they are able to control what exactly makes its way into the cell and what makes its way out of the cell.
- They provide structural components for the brain (roughly 60% of the brain is made of fatty acids). The primary fatty acid found in the brain is DHA, which you can get from eating foods high in Omega-3 fats.

- Vitamins A, D, E, and K are fat-soluble, meaning they must be dissolved in fat in order to be made bioavailable to the body.
- Fatty acids are the precursor for hormonal production by the
- endocrine system. If you aren't consuming enough fat, you may alter your metabolism by down-regulating endocrine function.
- Fat is extremely satiating and helps to regulate hunger cues.

| HOW MUCH DO YOU NEED

As with the first two macronutrients, we're beginning with the general guidelines so that you can get your fat to adequate and reasonable amounts to reap the benefits of a well-balanced dietary intake.

The general guideline for fat portions for women is as follows:

Using your thumb as a size guide, include one thumb-sized portion of fat-dense food with each meal, at least 4 times per day and no more than 6 times per day. If you are less active, keep to 4 servings, and if you are more active, increase to 5 or 6 portions.

Men:

Using your thumb as a size guide, include two thumb-sized portions of fat-dense food with each meal, at least four times a day. If you are less active, you can decrease your fat intake to a total of 6 servings each day.

| A NOTE ON UNSEEN FAT

Not all fat is visible on the plate. Cooking oil counts as fat intake, as does fat marbling in meat, and in the yokes of eggs. But please, don't stress over proper amounts in these unseen fat sources. We understand it's nearly impossible to figure out how much stir-fry to put on your plate if you only want to eat one thumbs-worth of cooking oil. If you know you have an oil-heavy dish or a fatty cut of meat, just be mindful of adding additional fat sources like avocado or nuts or dressings.

| HEALTH-SUPPORTING FAT-DENSE FOODS

- Avocados
- Olives and Olive Oil
- Coconut Oil
- Cheese and Full-Fat Unsweetened, Unflavored Dairy
- Whole Eggs
- Fatty Fish - Wild-Caught Salmon, Arctic Char, Atlantic Mackerel, and Black Cod to name a few
- Nuts
- Chia Seeds
- Ground Flax Seeds

| FAT TRAPS

It's worth mentioning that there are a couple of fat traps out there (foods that are healthy in moderation but extremely difficult to not over consume). The demonization of carbohydrates (restricted or eliminated) and glorification of fats (over-indulgent intake) has caused many to dramatically over consume calories (throwing their net energy balance out of whack). Or, worse, to create "franken-diets" (keeping the densely caloric fatty foods recommended by keto/paleo/carb-cycling gurus, but unable to consistently eliminate or restrict carbohydrate intake). All this to say, if you have spent years fearing carbohydrates be wary of excessive fat intake.

| FROM FEAR TO PEACE

> "Whatever you do, work heartily, as for the Lord and not for men, knowing that from the Lord you will receive the inheritance as your reward. You are serving the Lord Christ." Colossians 3: 23-24

Restoring our relationship with food back to its intended purpose—anchored in God's truth—is the foundation of this transformation journey. Once the process of transformation takes root, we must choose to walk alongside others, helping them break free from a life of servitude to diet culture, exposing its weapons: fear and the stronghold of shame.

We can no longer sit by and watch as friends, loved ones, and young people destroy their emotional and physical health through the worldly idol of chronic, cyclical dieting. Dieting's lure is fear of not measuring up, it controls through false guilt, and then imprisons its faithful by the enemy's stronghold of shame. We must be bold and stand firm because we battle a culture that is monolithic. It is a culture that captures hearts and minds through fixing our eyes on our flesh and the world. After years living in and for diet culture, identity is claimed and the truth of who we are--heirs to the Kingdom, beautiful, wonderfully and fearfully made, worthy, image bearers of God--is destroyed. Fear is a liar and temporary transformation is not worth our peace.

"The thief comes only to steal
and kill and destroy; I have
come that they may have life,
and have it to the full."

John 10:10

| UNWORTHY MASTERS LEAD TO DIS-EASE:

"Be not wise in your own eyes; fear the Lord, and
turn away from evil." Proverbs 3:7

Through misinformation and agenda-driven, "cherry-picked"
research, diet culture has undermined our trust in the foods God
provided and in our amazing bodies. We fear fruit, eggs, dairy,
animal protein, gluten, grain, and in some of the more dangerous
diets we are told to fear vegetables. We no longer trust our palates or
hear our bodies distinct signals of hunger or fullness. The majority
of us now have a toxic relationship with food and dislike our bodies
because we are lost in the seduction, never-ending confusion, and
fear mongering of diet culture. Our faith in diet culture, for even the
most deeply rooted Christian, has supplanted God's protection and
the peace only he provides. The truth:

- God's provision is perfectly designed to fuel our bodies
- Self-control is Spirit empowered, not willpowered
- Our strength to resist temptation comes from Christ alone

The solution to our growing health and weight issues seems to be
just plain common sense: return to God's truth. However, the enemy
has used diet culture well: false fear and shame have elevated the
importance of our flesh and moved our dependence in this area to
worldly wisdom, leaving us unprotected against the temptations of
both.

Eating, a necessary process, is now the focus of our thoughts and
actions. In a quest to look better and fear of whatever calamity
awaits us if we make the wrong food choice, diet culture dictates
our lifestyles. We worship certain foods (superfoods) and demonize
others (carbs are the enemy). We create false idols of worldly
"authorities". We grow increasingly self-reliant and self-loathing.

When we are temporarily successful, we celebrate our own strength. When we falter--and diet culture makes certain we falter--we add another brick in the stronghold of shame.

Make no mistake about it, diet culture is an asherah pole. Is it surprising that diet culture co-ops religious language? The heartbreak: diet culture is an unworthy master. It does not deserve our faith because it is destroying our wellness:

The price of faith in diet culture:

- The health and weight crisis is at epidemic proportions, growing worse each year despite decades of dieting (and now stealing our childrens' peace)
- Disordered and dysfunctional eating are rampant
- Diet culture's stronghold of shame continues to strengthen as it consumes hearts and minds
- Fellowship is pushed aside as we try to control our social and emotional situations
- Fellowship is destroyed through the dart of comparison
- Families lose relationship strengthening time around the dinner table because everyone's food restrictions make cooking a family meal arduous
- Intimate time with God is sacrificed in the constant toil of food fears and worries

God knew. But, despite his warning in Matthew 6:31-32 or his protection plan against false idols through the command to seek the Kingdom first in Matthew 6:33, we continue to empower diet culture. Our faith in this unworthy master has position God, at best, a distant third in our relationship with food and our bodies.

"So don't worry about these things, saying, 'What will we eat? What will we drink? What will we wear?' These things dominate the thoughts of unbelievers, but your heavenly Father already knows all your needs."

Matthew 6:31-32

| GOD'S TRUTH LEADS TO HIS PEACE:

These past weeks, you have begun the process to physically and emotionally transform your relationship with food through common sense nutrition and relying on God's goodness. Throughout this time, as your dependence on God has grown in this area, trust that he has been faithfully renewing your mind to free you from diet culture fear and restore your peace through his "good, pleasing, and perfect will."

Trust that God did not leave you alone in this battle against your flesh and the world. Run to his Word because the truth about food, its purpose and its proper place is woven throughout the Bible.

Just a few verses to put on the full armor of God against the unworthy master of diet culture:

- We are told food was designed for our good (Genesis 1:29, Genesis 9:3)
- We are told not to worship food (1 Cor 8:8; 1 Cor 6:12)
- We are made in God's image: loved and of such worth (Jer 31:3; Romans 5:8)
- We are cautioned not to abuse food and called to a narrow path of moderation and self-control (Phil 3:19; Prov 23:2; 1 Cor 6:19-20; Prov 25:16)

God's wisdom and desire for our good is so complete that He knew His peace would be desperately needed in this area:

> "For the kingdom of God is not a matter of eating
> and drinking, but of righteousness, peace and joy
> in the Holy Spirit," Romans 14:17

With a renewed mind, we can break free and be authentically transformed. Speak boldly against diet culture and strengthen each other in the truth. Allow God's transformative power to work through you and be a light for others still battling on this field. Be a light that is an example of how through Christ alone the desires of our flesh and the fear of the world are powerless. Remind others through the peace God have given you in your relationship with food and body that self-control is Spirit empowered and joy-filled; that fear is a liar:

When he told you you're not worthy When he
told you you're not loved When he told you
you're not beautiful That you'll never be enough

Fear, he is a liar
He will rob your rest
Steal your happiness

Cast your fear in the fire 'Cause fear he is a liar

Zach Williams

NOTES

AT THE KING'S TABLE

THAT'S THE GOOD STUFF

"When the report was heard in Pharaoh's house, "Joseph's brothers have come," it pleased Pharaoh and his servants. And Pharaoh said to Joseph, "Say to your brothers, 'Do this: load your beasts and go back to the land of Canaan, And take your father and your households, and come unto me: and I will give you the good of the land of Egypt, and ye shall eat the fat of the land."

Genesis 45:16-18

There's a reason bacon, a cut of meat that's at least 50% fat, has gained notoriety as one of America's favorite foods. Fat is the GOOD stuff! Fat adds wonderful and robust flavor to food, it enhances the satiety factor of food, it adds moisture and a tender texture to baked goods, it emulsifies ingredients in mixtures like dressings and marinades, and is incredibly effective at transferring heat in the cooking process, allowing us to have everything from deep-fried foods to stir-fry and sautes.

It's no wonder why the ancient cultures looked at fat as a luxury and gift from God. Genesis 45 is just one example of that ideal come to life. In this passage we see that Joseph's brothers - the ones who sold him into slavery out of sheer jealousy - coming to Egypt where Joseph served in the Pharoah's house. The Pharaoh, having respect for Joseph, celebrated their coming by promising them the fat of the land, or, in other words, all the best the land of Egypt has to offer.

Which makes us wonder, what is the fat of life? What adds a burst of flavor to your life? What adds weight and significance to your memories? Let's take the next 15 minutes to take time to point out all of the "fat" of life. Look high and low, finding all of your little hidden gems.

| LEADER-LED DISCUSSION:

- Give everyone 15 or so minutes to make a list of all of the fat of life. Encourage them to look beyond the obvious, like family members and friends

| THE FAT OF LIFE:

EUCHARISTEO

If you haven't yet, we recommend you go pick up a copy of Ann Voskamp's *One Thousand Gifts*. In this poetic book filled with Voskamp's personal experiences and insights, she delves into the heart of Eucharisteo, or the Greek word for the phrase, "he gave thanks." Finding this word to be interesting, she dives right in. As it turns out, the root word for Eucharisteo is *charis*, or the Greek word for "grace." And the derivative for *charis* is... ? *Chara*, or the Greek word for "joy."

So if we put all of this together we can see that the act of giving thanks taps into a divine grace that's rooted in an eternal joy.

Divine grace ... eternal joy... notice how both of these, both the divine and the eternal, are rooted in the supernatural which makes them independent of the natural. In other words, no matter what is happening in this worldly life, you have been given a tool that can reconnect you to the supernatural gifts of grace and joy. Next time your life turns upside down, say "thank you."

> *"The highest form of prayer is to the goodness of God... God only desires that our soul cling to him with all of its strength, in particular, that it clings to His goodness. For of all the things our minds can think about God, it is thinking upon His goodness that pleases Him most and brings the most profit to our soul."*
>
> *Julian of Norwich*

The fat of life, the good stuff that adds flavor and sustenance and holds everything together, is our anchor to a life lived in a state of Eucharisteo. Our problem is we go through life allowing our problems to cloud up our entire field of vision. Focusing on all that's bad, not all that's right, is like saying that you respect the size of your problem more than you respect the size of your solution: JESUS.

Keep the list you just made handy, referencing it often, to keep the goodness of God top of mind. We recommend keeping it near your Bible or journal so you can review it every time you sit down for a devotional or writing time.

"My soul shall be satisfied as with marrow and fatness; and my mouth shall praise thee with joyful lips." Psalm 63:5

| READING ASSIGNMENT

- Matthew 9

UNWORTHY MASTER

| LEADER-LED DISCUSSION:

How is "from fear to peace" coming along?

If needed, remind yourself and those walking this journey with you:

Diet culture is anchored in immediate gratification and a fast start. In fact, it is to their benefit when you get quick results. You become their best free marketing tool. When you falter—fall off the wagon—you still market for them: "It was great." "I felt so good." "I messed up or this happened, but when I was on track it worked so I am going to start again." Diets and lifestyles (can we just be honest: they are BOTH diets) rely on repeat customers. They prey on ,and deepen, our toxic relationship with food and our bodies. They KNOW you will, at some point, fall off the wagon and derail from your diet. Their goal is different from yours: they want you to quickly lose weight too. However, where you never want to gain it back, diet culture profits when you do. For diet culture, there is always another Monday, another New Year, and another low point in the dressing room. They are certain your dislike of your body and inability to adhere to their restrictive tactics will over-shadow your common sense: diets never work.

Diet culture creates one sustainable lifestyle: chronic, cyclical dieting.

| TWO MASTERS

> *"No one can serve two masters. Either you will hate the one and love the other, or you will be devoted to the one and despise the other. You cannot serve both God and money." Matthew 6:24*

God knew the battle in which we would find ourselves: between flesh and spirit; between our worldview and Kingdom mindset; between our way and His way. He knew our minds and hearts would be divided. He knew the enemy would relentlessly attack us through worldly culture and our human desires. He knew, if we were not fully surrendered to Him, that we would become enslaved by both; torn from His protection and peace. Matthew, Chapter 6, warns us against all that might tear us from God and teaches us the freedom of a Kingdom first life. Simply, Matthew 6, verse 24 instructs that it is impossible to be worldly and serve God. Jesus wants ALL of us. So, the choice: whom will you serve? That which enslaves you or the One who sets you free (2 Corinthians 5:17).

| LEADER-LED DISCUSSION:

- Why is it best to serve God and surrender our will to His?
- What is your experience when you fall prey to your own desires or the ways of the world?
- What happens in any circumstance where you shift your focus from self/world to God?

| OBEDIENCE

> "Don't you know that when you offer yourselves to someone as obedient slaves, you are slaves of

the one you obey — whether you are slaves to
sin, which leads to death, or to obedience, which
leads to righteousness?" Romans 6:16

Obedience to God always brings blessings. We are hard-wired to
know this truth and immediately feel the peace of obedient choices;
however, we also live in a fallen world and are a rebellious lot. Often,
we are not aware if we are being obedient to God's will for our lives
or imposing our own desires. So, first, we must understand the
Biblical definition of obedience.

In the Old Testament, obedience—when used in relationship to
God— is "to hear," "to listen" with reverence to a greater authority.
In the New Testament, the concept of obedience takes on greater
spiritual significance. In Eerdmans Bible Dictionary, Christian
obedience is defined beautifully:

"True 'hearing,' or obedience, involves the physical hearing that
inspires the hearer, and a belief or trust that in turn motivates the
hearer to act in accordance with the speaker's desires."

New Testament Biblical obedience is fully trusting that God's will
for our lives is better. To obey is to surrender to Him and to His
Word; it is to live a life walking closely with God. When we walk
closely with God and choose to be in an intimate relationship with
Him—through time in His Word, our prayers, worship and praise—
then we are able to discern His will from our own. We are able
to know His voice and hear the Holy Spirit's guidance. We are
better able to separate His plan and purpose for our lives from our
own desires. Our focus shifts from toiling for a desired outcome
to the peace and assurance of a fully surrendered life. An obedient
Christian let's go and then let's God.

We live confident in His Truth and obediently serve his will. Despite discomfort, doubt, or fear we know His plan is better. We know that our best life brings Him glory. An obedient Christian immerses themselves in His Word, running to Him first in every circumstance. We ask: God how can this circumstance be used for your glory? How can your purpose be best served? God will never forsake his chosen; He is, by his nature: faithful. He did not abandon us to figure things out on our own in this fallen world. Rather, when we passionately study the Bible, His plan and purpose for our lives is revealed. We begin to see where God is in the midst of our circumstance. We begin to hear his desires for us over our own or the world's. The more passionately we surrender to God's wisdom, the more attuned we are to His Spirit; the greater our discernment.

Obedience unleashes the Spirit's power to renew and transform. An obedient life, where we desire to serve only God, produces rich fruit: peace, love, grace, forgiveness, and freedom.

LEADER-LED DISCUSSION:

- Paul writes in Romans 6:17 "But thanks be to God that, though you *used* to be slaves to sin, you have come to obey from your heart the pattern of teaching that has now claimed your allegiance." He writes in the past tense because YOU HAVE BEEN FREED when you put your faith in Christ. In what areas of your life are you choosing to enslave yourself by obeying your own desires or following the world's way?

BLESSINGS

"But whoever looks intently into the perfect law that gives freedom, and continues in it—not

> forgetting what they have heard, but doing it—
> they will be blessed in what they do." James 1:25

As we learned in Matthew 6, we simply cannot serve two masters. We must choose to serve our own desires or live to fulfill God's purpose for our lives. Obedience is not knowing God's Truth; it is choosing to act in accordance with it. God's grace and Christ's obedience wiped us clean, enabling us to live eternally with our Heavenly Father. However, during our time on mission in this fallen world, obedience is the way to experience "all the things" promised in Matthew 6:33. An obedient life keeps our eyes fixed on Jesus: all the abundance we will ever need and far more than we deserve. Obedience allows the Holy Spirit to renew and transform us so that we can experience God's promises:

> "For the kingdom of God is not a matter of eating
> and drinking, but of righteousness, peace and joy
> in the Holy Spirit, because anyone who serves
> Christ in this way is pleasing to God and receives
> human approval. Let us therefore make every
> effort to do what leads to peace and to mutual
> edification." Romans 14:17-19

Obediently serving God is true freedom. It frees us from our destructive desires through the strength of Christ. As well, obediently serving God with everything we are releases us from the grip of worry (Matthew 6:25). Ignited faith, wholly lived out, blesses us with a peace that surpasses all understanding and one that is not dependent on our temporary circumstance. An obedient life results in a cup that is not only full, but one that overflows. Only through our obedience can we know true satisfaction (Leviticus 26:3-10). One need only look to Jesus to see a perfect example of humble obedience and its fruit. God's call for us to be obedient does not grow out of a desire to enslave; rather, our obedience liberates us and leads to LIFE.

| LEADER-LED DISCUSSION:

- Do you trust that serving Christ obediently, surrendering to God fully, leads to freedom in ALL areas of your life?
- Do you serve God in a way that recognizes that He gives and that you need Him? In other words, is your service from the fruit of the Holy Spirit; service that turns its back on self-reliance?
- Discuss how building an intimate relationship with God is above all other needs.

CONCLUSION

| LEADER-LED DISCUSSION:

- Open the floor to questions and ending discussion; set time cap if needed
- Close in specific prayer for each area in which surrender is needed and take a moment to give thanks for this journey

| READING ASSIGNMENTS

Romans 6:16
Deuteronomy 11:26-28
Psalm 103
Luke 5
Matthew 22:36-38
John 14:15

"For the kingdom of God is not a matter of eating and drinking, but of righteousness, peace and joy in the Holy Spirit, because anyone who serves Christ in this way is pleasing to God and receives human approval. Let us therefore make every effort to do what

Romans 14:17-19

FINAL NOTE: MAKE GOD THE GREATEST DESIRE OF YOUR HEART

"When tempted, no one should say, "God is tempting me." For God cannot be tempted by evil, nor does he tempt anyone;but each person is tempted when they are dragged away by their own evil desire and enticed. Then, after desire has conceived, it gives birth to sin; and sin, when it is full-grown, gives birth to death. Don't be deceived, my dear brothers and sisters. Every good and perfect gift is from above, coming down from the Father of the heavenly lights, who does not change like shifting shadows. He chose to give us birth through the word of truth, that we might be a kind of firstfruits of all he created." James 1:13-18

BREAK THROUGH is a six week journey to seek authentic transformation in your relationship with food and your body. It is time to plant seeds in rich soil. A time to acknowledge and demolish diet culture strongholds. A time to run to Jesus and prayerfully ask for conviction in this area of your life. Yes, we include nutrition information, but it is common sense. Our nutrition information doesn't require "diet culture, cherry-picked research" because it isn't founded in fear, trends, or rooted in confirmation bias. Rather, it is found in God's unchanging truth: from Genesis to Revelation.

Where diet culture calls us to faith in our own strength and to seek worldly knowledge in our desire for transformation, as believers we know the transformation the world offers is temporary. We know true transformation is God-sparked and Spirit led. We understand that until our minds are renewed, our flesh and the world will continue to imprison us in enemy strongholds. We understand it is only when we fix our eyes on Jesus and surrender completely that we experience the peace and joy of God. Romans 12:2 transformation is found in Christ alone. His strength alone demolishes strongholds. His truth alone transforms our thoughts, words, and actions so that our lives produce good fruit and bring glory to God.

Lay your relationship with food and your body at the foot of Cross. Truly. Run to God's Word and pray to seek His will. Allow the Holy Spirit to renew your mind and transform the desires of your heart. Be empowered to break free from diet culture and its strongholds of willpower, false guilt, and shame to the loving, grace-filled protection, freedom, and peace of God.

Remember: God provided everything we need to fuel our bodies and armed us with Biblical truth to guard against temptation. God calls us to honor our bodies without falling prey to self-worship so that we can glorify Him. He teaches us self-control through Spirit empowerment to protect us from willfulness and false idols.

We pray you MAKE GOD YOUR GREATEST DESIRE and bless Him with all that is within you:

> "Bless the Lord, O my soul, and all that is within me, bless his holy name!
>
> Bless the Lord, O my soul, and forget not all his benefits, who forgives all your iniquity, who heals all your diseases, who redeems your life from the pit, who crowns you with steadfast love and mercy, who satisfies you with good so that your youth is renewed like the eagle's." Psalm 103-1-5

Why does God deserve your constant, yielded faith-filled praise? He deserves all that is within you because of His Nature: He is unchanging and faithful. His love is steadfast and perfect. He is righteous and all-knowing.

He is good.

But God loves you so that He goes beyond who He is and gives you more:

> He FORGIVES
> He HEALS
> He REDEEMS
> He CROWNS
> He SATISFIES

His love for you is so unfailing that he gave his only Son:

> "The Lord is compassionate and gracious, slow to anger, abounding in love.

He will not always accuse, nor will he harbor his anger forever;

he does not treat us as our sins deserve or repay us according to our iniquities.

For as high as the heavens are above the earth, so great is his love for those who fear him; as far as the east is from the west, so far has he removed our transgressions from us..." Psalm 103: 8-12

Make God the greatest desire of your heart because of:

Who He is.
All He gives.
What Jesus did.

When you make God the greatest desire of your heart strongholds will fall and you will be abundantly filled.

Thank you for making us a part of your journey. You are always in our prayers.

Romans 12:2,

CAROL + ALEX

"Therefore, brothers and sisters, we have an obligation—but it is not to the flesh, to live according to it. For if you live according to the flesh, you will die; but if by the Spirit you put to death the misdeeds of the body, you will live."

"What, then, shall we say in response to these things? If God is for us, who can be against us? He who did not spare his own Son, but gave him up for us all—how will he not also, along with him, graciously give us all things?"

Romans 8: 12-14, 31-33

ABOUT THE AUTHORS:

CAROL BEVIL: personal trainer, nutrition coach, author, and speaker is co-founder of Fuel Your Body, Feed Your Soul, a God-first approach to nutrition, body image, and food relationship. She's been in the health and fitness industry for thirty years. She holds multiple certifications in personal training, cycling, and nutrition. Raised in a Jewish family, she surrendered her life to Jesus and was baptized with her husband at the age of forty. They have a son and three daughters and live in Birmingham, Alabama. Carol can be frequently found in her kitchen, cooking, drinking coffee, reading her Bible and writing.

Her life verse: Matthew 6:33

*　　*　　*

ALEX BRIGHAM:

A farm-raised Tennessee girl, Alex holds multiple certifications in personal training, nutrition and holistic lifestyle coaching. She was raised by two active and health-minded parents and found work in the health and fitness industry to be a natural fit. Growing up in the millennial generation, Alex experienced first-hand the damage of the modern lifestyle diets combined with the negative influence of social media. She has dedicated her life's work to helping others find a life of freedom from the diet mentality and from fear-driven restriction.

She lives by these words of Paul:

Romans 8:37-39: No, in all these things we are more than conquerors through him who loved us. For I am convinced that neither death nor life, neither angels nor demons, neither the present nor the future, nor any powers, neither height nor depth, nor anything else in all creation, will be able to separate us from the love of God that is in Christ Jesus our Lord.

For More Carol + Alex:

INSTA: @ FUELBODYFEEDSOUL
BLOG: WWW.FUELBODYFEEDSOUL.COM

OTHER BOOKS:

YOU ARE HIS: CLAIMING WHO YOU ARE
BECAUSE OF WHOSE YOU ARE (AVAILABLE
ON AMAZON AND BARNES & NOBLE)

Printed in Great Britain
by Amazon